A Guide to
Clinical Placements
in
Speech and Language
Therapy

Library of Congress Cataloguing in Publication Data

British Library Cataloguing in Publication Data

A catalogue record for this book is available from the British Library

Cover design: Jim Wilkie

Project management, typesetting and design: J&R Publishing Services Ltd, Guildford, Surrey, UK; www.jr-publishingservices.co.uk

A Guide to
Clinical Placements
in
Speech and Language
Therapy

Jennifer Louise Read

J&R Press Ltd

Printed and bound by CPI Group (UK) Ltd, Croydon, CR0 4YY

Contents

Foreword

Clinical placements are perhaps the most memorable aspect of studying to become a speech and language therapist. No matter how experienced the clinician, they are able to recall memories of dedicated clinical educators, inspirational clients and the rewarding feeling that comes when a client begins to make progress. They also remember the fear of clinical exams, trekking from bus stop to clinic in the snow, and the challenges of combining such a demanding and unique degree with student life. Clinical placements play a pivotal role in guiding students towards their future career. The huge range of specialisms in speech and language therapy mean that most students will have placements that inspire and motivate, and others that are simply not a good 'fit'. The relationship between a student and their clinical educator can make or break a placement. There are a great many factors at play in the overall success of a placement in the student's eyes.

Over the last 10 years, I have made the transition from a student studying speech and language therapy at university to a senior lecturer in speech and language therapy. Hearing the current students' tales of their experiences on placement brought the memories of my own student days flooding back, but I also realised how valuable these accounts could be for those about to embark on their own journey to become a practising speech and language therapist. There is an abundance of textbooks designed to help students understand the theoretical underpinnings and evidence-base of working with clients, but little has been written from a student perspective about the realities of being on a clinical placement. This book aims to fill that gap, enabling students to gain insight into the real-life experiences of placement from students who have been in that position. It is hoped that this book could be a useful source for prospective students who are deciding whether to apply to university. For those already studying to become a speech and language therapist, the chapters may provide a useful guide in terms of identifying particular placements of interest, or to prepare for a forthcoming placement with one of the client groups discussed. It is anticipated that this book will be an additional source for pre-placement preparation, alongside lectures, seminars and other published sources. I also hope that it will be of some value to academic staff and clinical educators, perhaps as a reminder of how we all felt as a student about to embark on our clinical placements.

Organising the chapters according to client group was a somewhat difficult decision. Much of the emphasis in clinical education is, quite rightly, on the development of transferable clinical skills. This encourages students to recognise that many of the skills they develop can be applied to a range of different clients, allowing them to work competently across client groups. Chapter 3 recognises the importance of transferable skills and it is highly recommended that all students read this chapter because it has relevance to every one of their clinical placements. However, when students are allocated placements, they are typically given information about the location and client group. Because this is a practical resource designed to aid students in their placement preparation, the book has been organised in stand-alone chapters which relate to the most common client groups seen by speech and language therapists within the UK.

It has been a privilege to talk to so many students about their experiences on placement. Without exception, they have been candid, enthusiastic and insightful. This book is dedicated to all of those students, and to the many more who are about to embark on such a unique and rewarding journey.

Jen Read
October 2013

1 Clinical education for speech and language therapy students

Speech and language therapists (SLTs) have specific expertise in working with people who have speech, language, communication and swallowing impairments. Graduate SLTs are qualified to work with a wide range of clients across a breadth of different health, education and legal settings. Clients range in age from neonatal to elderly and also vary enormously in terms of their difficulties. In short, qualified SLTs have a vast range of skills and areas of expertise and must undertake a challenging and exciting degree programme to equip themselves for professional practice.

Speech and language therapy is in its relative infancy compared to other medical and allied health professions. From the early days of a national diploma in SLT, there are now an increasing number of universities that offer recognised graduate and postgraduate degree courses which allow professional registration upon successful completion. In the United Kingdom, students undertake a 3–4-year undergraduate degree, or a 2-year master's degree. Courses leading to professional registration must be accredited by the Health and Care Professions Council (HCPC) and the Royal College of Speech and Language Therapists (RCSLT). Both the HCPC and RCSLT have detailed sets of professional standards that all graduates must meet in order to practise as a speech and language therapist in the UK. Training to become an SLT involves the study of a wide range of foundation subject areas: linguistics, phonetics, education science, biomedical sciences and psychology. These foundations are built upon with more specific training about speech, language, communication and swallowing disorders in a range of paediatric and adult populations.

Clinical education is a mandatory element of all speech and language therapy degree programmes. Graduates must possess both the theoretical knowledge and practical skills to enable safe, effective and professional practice. Lectures, seminars, tutorials, problem-based learning and clinical placements are all used to develop the crucial professional and clinical skills required by graduate SLTs in order to practise. In the early stages of most degrees, university-based teaching is centred on the theoretical underpinnings of clinical work. A range of core transferable skills is often the focus of these sessions, which include goal setting, writing case notes, session planning and many other practical skills. Problem-based learning is also becoming a more common mode of delivery, whereby students begin to apply the theory to clinical cases within the safe confines of the classroom environment.

Placements during the early stages are often heavily weighted towards observation. Students gain experience through observing an expert clinician at work and, of course, observing client behaviour. Some institutions have campus clinics which provide a safe and well-supervised model for clinical education during the initial stages of practice. Students are encouraged to take on a more autonomous role as they progress through their studies, and the number of placement hours usually increases with each year of the course. Universities and the clinical community collaborate to provide students with a supportive learning environment in which to learn and develop their clinical skills. Effective clinical education relies on the commitment of the student, academic staff and experienced clinicians. Clinical educators facilitate, supervise and manage practice-based learning and help students to apply their knowledge to practice in real-world contexts. As such, the relationship between students and their clinical educators is crucial to the overall success of a placement.

Research into the perspectives of clinical educators has revealed a number of student characteristics that clinical educators hold in high regard. Willingness to engage and learn, professional behaviour, and personal attributes such as honesty, empathy and taking initiative have all been rated extremely highly by clinical educators in the allied health professions (Chipchase et al., 2012). These attributes were rated more highly than knowledge, understanding and skills, suggesting perhaps that transferable skills such as these are critical from the start of a placement whereas some of the knowledge and skills pertaining to a specific client group can be acquired during the course of particular placements. Pre-clinical teaching at university and an understanding of clinical educators' expectations may go some way towards easing the anxiety that most students experience prior to clinical placements.

Clinical placements aim to facilitate the transferral of knowledge into practice and allow students to apply what they have learned in the classroom to real contexts and clients. McAllister et al. state that "clinical education is about the real world of professional practice where learning is holistic and involves transfer, reorganisation, application, synthesis and evaluation of previously acquired knowledge" (McAllister, Lincoln, McLeod, & Maloney,

1997). It is also important to recognise that clinical educators often benefit enormously from student supervision. Clinicians report satisfaction in being able to share their expertise and in seeing their student develop over the course of a placement (Dilbert & Goldenberg, 1995). They also benefit from students bringing fresh ideas and recent evidence-based practice into their service, which can enhance their own practice.

An international perspective

Alongside university-based lectures, seminars and tutorials, all students are required to undertake clinical placements. In the UK, students are required to complete 150 sessions of clinical placement, 100 of which must be directly supervised by a qualified speech and language therapist (Joint Accreditation Committee of the HPC and the RCSLT, 2002). The guidelines stipulate that over the course of their degree programme, students must experience a range of clinical settings and types of service delivery, as well as working with clients who range in age and complexity and present with difficulties stemming from a range of aetiologies. The majority of graduate courses are structured to provide a combination of weekly and block placements and students are usually allocated one or more experienced speech and language therapists to supervise their clinical work and provide expert guidance.

Speech and language therapy is a growing international profession, with an increasing number of services and education providers worldwide. Whilst the courses leading to clinical qualification do differ, all students must meet high standards of proficiency and undertake clinical placements in order to gain their qualification. For example, whilst the number of clinical hours is not stipulated by Speech Pathology Australia, students must demonstrate that they have met a detailed set of competencies (Speech Pathology Speech Pathology Australia, 2011). The American Speech-Language-Hearing Association (ASHA) specify that students must complete 400 supervised hours of clinical education within a range of settings and with a variety of clinical populations. The NetQues report examined speech and language therapy education in 31 European countries, reporting that students from all institutions are required to undertake a minimum number of external clinical hours, ranging from 70 to 1360 hours (Csefalvay et al., 2013). These selected examples illustrate the wide range of requirements stipulated internationally, though it must also be recognised that most individual degree courses require students to undertake many more hours of clinical practice than these minimum standards specify.

Although the standards leading to accreditation vary internationally, some countries are part of an agreement known as the Mutual Recognition of Professional Association Credentials (MRA). The agreement between six national associations came into force in 2009, and allows registered members of one association to be recognised by another in some cases. The MRA suggests that there is sufficient commonality between qualifying courses and the profession in the UK, Ireland, Australia, the United States, New Zealand and Canada to allow some degree of mutual recognition.

How to use this book

Clinical placements are an integral part of training to become a speech and language therapist. Most students find them the most anxiety-provoking aspect of their studies, yet also the most stimulating and engaging element of their degree course. Placements set vocational degrees apart from other degree-level education, providing students with experience of the workplace that they hope to enter upon completion of their studies. Most students gain insight into their forthcoming placements from reading, lectures, university staff, and their clinical educator. Whilst these are all valuable sources for information and guidance, students often feel underprepared for the day-to-day realities of placement and many turn to their peers for understanding and support. This book aims to give students a voice and act as another 'peer' to provide them with a deeper understanding of the challenges and rewards they are likely to experience. Chapter 2 outlines the methodology of the book, detailing the procedure and participants involved. Chapter 3 examines the transferable skills required across all placements irrespective of the clients encountered. Chapters 4 to 12 can be read independently of one another. Each chapter aims to provide an insight into working with the most common client groups that students encounter when on clinical placements in the UK. Each chapter is organised according to key themes, and contains advice for students from both their peers and from clinical educators working in the particular specialist areas of practice. Chapter 13 offers a summary of the study and examines the future of clinical education.

2 Methodology

Focus group

The study began with a focus group facilitated by the author, attended by five students in the final year of their undergraduate degree in speech and language therapy. The students were invited to discuss their recent block placement, giving a brief summary of their experiences, highlighting their initial expectations of the placement and the challenges they faced. They were then asked to consider the premise of this text in the context of their own experiences throughout the degree programme.

Perhaps surprisingly, the students felt that the focus group was the first time that they had discussed their own placement experiences in-depth with their peers, and they found this a very positive learning experience. They often had little contact with their peers during the course of a block placement and, due to confidentiality, were unable to discuss many aspects of their work. The qualitative nature of the study was positively received. The students felt that they would be able to relate to the accounts and experiences of other students and that it would be useful to present these perspectives in an accessible style. Rather than feeling that the detailed and honest accounts of placement would provoke anxiety, the students felt that they would be reassured and better prepared as a result of reading about other students' experiences.

Participants

Students were recruited from two universities in the United Kingdom. Information about the type of placement that each student had just completed was used to select the students approached for the study in order to gain information about working with a wide range of client groups. The students were emailed with information about the study and they contacted the researcher if they wanted to consent to take part. Fifty-two interviews were carried out with a total of 44 students. Eight students had been on a 'split placement', working with two different client groups and so were interviewed twice. All of the students were in their final year of their undergraduate degree in speech and language therapy, and had completed a block placement with the particular client group within six weeks of the interview taking place. The students were also asked to complete a proforma listing their 'top five tips' to students about to embark on placement with the same client group.

Practising speech and language therapists were also asked to state their 'top five tips' for prospective students working with their client group. All of the SLTs were experienced clinical educators who had supervised students on placement within the last 12 months. Letters and emails were sent to 72 speech and language therapists, followed up three weeks later with another email and letter to those who had not responded to the initial request for information. The response rate was 74%.

Conduct of the study followed procedures approved by Manchester Metropolitan University's Faculty Ethics Committee (Ref: 1129). Written, informed consent was gained from each student participant.

Interviews and transcription

Following consent, the student interviews were conducted either face-to-face or over the telephone by the author, and ranged in length from 24 to 58 minutes. The in-depth, semi-structured interviews were based around five key questions, which were formulated following analysis of the focus group transcripts to identify key themes. Approximately one week prior to the interview, the list of topic areas was sent to the students and they were asked to spend some time considering their experiences in the context of these topics. The five core questions were:

1. What were the specific challenges of working with the client group?

2. Were there any unexpected aspects of the experience?

3. Were there any emotional impacts related to working with this client group?

4. Can you reflect on the specific environment in which you spent your placement?

5. Can you tell me about the your role as a speech and language therapy student with the client group?

Responses that did not directly address the stimuli questions were included to add depth and novel responses to the study. All interviews were audio-recorded using a digital voice recorder and then subsequently transcribed verbatim. Any data that breached confidentiality in terms of identifying people or places were removed from the transcripts. The students were briefed prior to the interview that the interviews would focus on their personal experiences on placement, and that they should avoid discussing specific people or locations.

Data coding and analysis

The transcripts for each client group were all read closely and repeatedly prior to being loaded separately according to client group into QSR NVivo 8 in order for data analysis to be conducted according to client group. Data were analysed by a thematic analysis approach using thematic networks (Attride-Stirling, 2001) in NVivo. Any identifying information was removed from the transcripts to maintain confidentiality and anonymity of the students, agencies, places and clients. In each chapter, the data are presented and organised according to the 'global themes' that arose from the analysis. In some cases, there are additional subthemes which separate some of the global themes into distinct topics. Each chapter presents a background to the client group and a brief theoretical context. The qualitative data form the main component of each chapter, providing a unique insight into the students' experiences. All of the names used are pseudonyms. The 'top tips' which complete each chapter were compiled from the students interviewed for each particular chapter, and from clinicians working with clients and students in each specific clinical context.

3 Transferable clinical skills

One of the core challenges facing education in speech and language pathology is aligning the curriculum with the evolving knowledge base about communication disorders and the changing contexts in which new graduates are employed. Whether the curriculum should be driven by client-specific knowledge or transferable skills remains a matter for debate, though it is acknowledged that most universities address this dichotomy by teaching both specific and transferable skills (Brumfitt, Enderby, & Hoben, 2005). Thus, new graduates are able to work effectively with different client groups in a range of contexts. There is no guidance as to the types of clinical placements that students are required to undertake during their degree. The UK guidelines stipulate experience with a 'wide range' of client groups and the development of transferable skills which allow graduates to practise competently in a range of different contexts. The emphasis on transferable skills is perhaps becoming more pertinent in the changing healthcare and education climates. Previously, new graduates often took on a mixed adult and paediatric caseload upon graduation; however, these 'split posts' are becoming increasingly rare and new graduates are securing more specialist roles. The challenge for universities is to design a curriculum that enables students to gain sufficient specialist knowledge and skills whilst equipping all graduates with the abilities needed to work with an ever-increasing range of clients.

What is a 'good' speech and language therapist?

There is relatively little research into the skills and qualities that make for an effective speech and language therapist, leading to some lack of insight for educators in terms of how best to prepare students for both placements and employment beyond. There is, however, a growing body of literature about the skills that speech and language therapy service managers regard highly in newly qualified SLTs. In a study by Brumfitt et al. (2005), managers identified four key qualities that they felt an 'ideal' therapist should possess: good communicator, good practioner, good person and good administrator.

These labels encompassed many generic skills such as time management and staying organised. Interestingly, most of the specific traits highlighted were personal qualities and highly transferable across client groups. Being flexible and conscientious, having negotiation and listening skills and keeping accurate records were all deemed to be important, though as Brumfitt et al. (2005) debate, many of these skills are difficult to teach within the constraints of university. Rather, it is important that prospective students already possess some of these traits prior to beginning their studies and develop them further as they acquire clinical experience during their speech and language therapy degree. Stansfield (2001, cited in Stansfield, 2004) also examined the personal traits that were considered important qualities for a speech and language therapist to possess and found that being enthusiastic, hard-working and motivated were highly desirable. Students interviewed for the same study felt that they gained most from working with clinical educators who were passionate about their work. A recent large-scale European study examined responses from nearly 5000 employers, recent graduates and academics about the areas of practice in which newly-qualified therapists should be able to demonstrate competence (Csefalvay et al., 2013). There was a high level of agreement between all three groups surveyed, who felt that being able to assess, diagnose and implement appropriate therapy were all critical skills. The results also showed that understanding professional roles boundaries and making appropriate referrals to other agencies were also highly desirable. The study also revealed that generic competencies such as empathy, honesty, self-reflection and sensitivity were valued highly. These studies all suggest that a great deal is expected from students and newly-qualified therapists; however, many of the core requirements relate to personal qualities and forging relationships with colleagues and clients as opposed to the more specific skills that new graduates often worry about.

The importance of clinical education

Clinical placements are an integral part of all qualifying degree courses. Although there are individual differences between courses, all students are required to demonstrate their clinical skills with a range of client populations and demonstrate to their clinical educators and academic tutors that they are able to work safely and effectively. The importance of clinical education is not only acknowledged by educators but also by students and newly-qualified therapists themselves. Brumfitt et al. (2005) asked newly-qualified therapists (NQTs) to review the elements of their degree courses that they felt best prepared them for working life. The results showed that placements were rated far more highly than any other aspect, with 81% of NQTs identifying clinical experience as the most important component of their course. More specifically, they felt that having their sessions observed by their clinical educator whilst on placement was the most useful learning experience. The NQTs stressed the importance of building good working relationships with their clinical educators and felt that their CEs were fundamental in terms of building up or knocking their confidence. Block placements were perceived to help build confidence and were considered to be the most representative of real working life. In a 2001 study by Stansfield (cited in Stansfield, 2004), clinical educators, students and university academics were asked to reflect on the process of clinical education for speech and language therapy students. The outcomes could be summarised according to three broad themes: competence and clinical knowledge, clinical skill and personal characteristics. Knowledge and theory were deemed to be important and placements were seen as integral to the application of acquired knowledge into practice. A wide range of technical clinical skills were highlighted, all of which were transferable across client groups, for example problem solving, making client referrals, analysing data and many other technical competencies. Flexibility was one of the most important clinical skills highlighted by all three groups of participants in the study, who suggested that being able to adapt to individual client's needs was one of the critical factors that influenced the overall success of a therapy session. The students interviewed for the present study also identified flexibility as a core skill. Producing session plans with inbuilt contingency strategies and working with a client according to their needs and behaviours on a particular day were themes within student's reflections that rose in interviews about working with every client group.

> I think it's really challenging, really challenging…the kids are not necessarily going to do what you want them to do. So it's you that needs to be flexible, that's the main thing. Be very, very flexible. **Jade**

Stansfield (2004) also reported that many students lacked confidence in their clinical skills and that academics and supervising clinicians were well aware of the anxiety that most students feel about their clinical placements. The forthcoming chapters show that although many of the students were extremely nervous immediately prior to placement, their confidence in terms of working with clients increased tremendously as they gained experience throughout their placements.

> I went in feeling absolutely terrified...I was trying to read everything I could possibly read...I was nervous about trying to remember everything...I was still nervous about just having conversation. **Richard**

'I didn't sleep for a week'...Why do clinical placements provoke such anxiety?

Students have always found clinical placements to be one of the most anxiety-provoking elements of their degree, though often the most enjoyable in practice. Research suggests that anxiety levels are highest prior to the first clinical experience in the early stages of study, but students in their final year also report high anxiety about placements (Chan, Carter, & McAllister, 1994). Unsurprisingly, students in their first year were nervous about their lack of experience in clinical settings and were concerned about managing their academic work alongside clinical placement. The first-year students were also observed to have very high expectations of their own performance and were keen to make a good impression on both their clinical educator and their clients. Perhaps more surprising were the findings that students in their final year were almost as nervous about their placement as the first-year students in the study (Chan et al., 1994). These findings are slightly at odds with the concept of a competent 'entry-level' student. Their fears about diagnosing and managing clients had been replaced with concerns about their competence to work professionally as they neared completion of their course. Certainly, some of the final-year students interviewed for this book were worried about their capacity to work autonomously and many lacked confidence in their own abilities. However, there were a number of other causes of anxiety linked specifically to the placement that they had just completed. In particular, the students who reported feeling the most nervous about their final placement were those who worked with a 'new' client group, that is, a client group that they had no practical experience of working with on previous placements. Some had never worked on a hospital ward before, others had little prior experience of talking to young children. For some of the students, this was their first experience of working closely with other professionals, or communicating with clients who used augmentative and alternative communication. Many of the students felt that these new clinical situations called into question the basic, transferable skills that they had already developed and held the belief that working with a new client group would feel like 'starting all over again'. The perceived expectation that clinical educators would expect students in the final stages of their studies to be competent and able to work autonomously was a major concern for many of the students on final-year placements. In reality, once they had embarked upon their 'new' placement, many of the students agreed that it was not as unfamiliar and daunting as they had expected. With support from their clinical educator, most students were quickly able to use the skills that they had acquired on previous placements and went on to achieve high marks. Chan et al. (1994) reported that assessment was also a key anxiety-provoking factor for final-year students and this was also a real concern for many students interviewed for this book. Many had become increasingly anxious about their final degree classifications and felt that their final placement marks were a reflection on their competence to practise following graduation.

In the early stages of a speech and language pathology degree, the students have relatively comparable levels of knowledge and clinical skill. As they progress through the years, each student builds up a portfolio of different clinical placements, which can sometimes lead to a perception that there is a lack of equity in the experience that students are gaining when compared with their peers. For instance, a student who has had several placements in a school for children with special needs may be perceived by their peers to be at an advantage in final clinical exams if they were to be placed in a similar context. Many of the students interviewed felt that if they were on this type of placement for the first time, they would be expected to reach the same clinical standards and marks would be awarded according to the same criteria as the student with more direct clinical experience. These discrepancies not only become more common as the students progress through the years, but they become more significant as students put increasing amounts of pressure on themselves to succeed and prove their capabilities.

The amount of experience was not the only factor cited by students as a perceived source of disparity and anxiety. Some considered particular client groups to be more challenging to work with and others felt that the restrictions of their particular placement had not allowed them to demonstrate the breadth of their knowledge and skills. This was a particular issue for students who spent much of their placement observing clients working with their clinical educator as opposed to actively carrying out sessions, or for students who experienced a high rate of non-attendance of clients.

Further research is required to ascertain whether these concerns are borne out by the clinical marks awarded to students at the end of placement. However, it is also critical that clinical educators and academic staff help students to see the wider picture. Clinical marks are no doubt important, but they represent one element of a multi-faceted degree programme, across which all students will have areas of strength and weakness. Gaining a wide range of clinical experience prior to qualification is invaluable and often the only opportunity to work with particular client groups in a long career. Students who work with a wide range of clients during their degree arguably gain a more diverse set of skills and are able to draw upon these experiences when making decisions about their future career and applying for posts following graduation. A student's employability might also be enhanced if they can demonstrate knowledge and experience across a breadth of areas. Clinical placements provide a rich learning environment that all students should embrace and enjoy, ensuring that they embark on each new experience with an open mind.

> I was actually quite excited about having that placement, because I think when you're on placement it's great to see as much as you can. And especially when you're a student you're still guided and supported by someone else. I tried to use all of the opportunities that I could to gain experience.
> **Martina**

The clinical journey

Most students begin their university journey with very limited experience of a speech and language therapy environment. Some will have shadowed a therapist prior to applying for their degree, others will have gained some experience by working in schools or nursing homes. The interviews conducted with students in their final year for this book suggest that nerves prior to embarking on a new placement never completely disappear, though the students' feelings and particular concerns do evolve over the course of their degree. Students passing through these stages have been described as 'novice', 'intermediate' and 'entry level' (McAllister & Lincoln, 2004). Students undertaking their first clinical placement are usually extremely anxious about interacting with clients and making a good impression on their clinical educator. Their concerns focus much more on their own performance than their clients' wellbeing at this stage, and they usually require a great deal of support from their clinical educators. My own personal experience in supporting students through their early placements suggests that many spend a great deal of time working on session plans and making resources, and often holding concerns about how much of their clinical educator's time they are 'taking up'. In fact, McAllister and Lincoln (2004) reported that supervising students at this early stage in their development can be extremely rewarding for clinical educators because of the significant progress often made by 'novice' students. 'Intermediate' students begin to reflect on their own performance, their client's performance and the interaction between these two factors (McAllister & Lincoln, 2004). Students are often given a higher degree of autonomy but continue to work closely with their clinical educator and access support in terms of clinical reasoning and linking theory to practice. During the late stages of their training, most students are able to work competently with far less support from their clinical educator, particularly if the clients are not too complex, and often the relationship between student and clinical educator becomes more collaborative rather than hierarchical.

Transferable skills

Very few of the students discussed 'transferable skills' in those terms specifically, though many did refer to particular skills that they felt crossed over their work with different client groups when they were asked specifically to reflect on transferable skills. There may be a number of explanations for this discrepancy. Firstly, some of the students may have lacked insight or confidence about their own skill set, or had never considered their skills in terms of being 'transferable'. Secondly, some of the students appeared to attach limited value to skills that are considered transferable and felt that much more kudos (and higher marks) could be gained from demonstrating more specific skills towards the end of their degree. Skills such as writing session plans and case notes, building rapport and working in a multidisciplinary team were often regarded by the students as basic skills mastered in the earlier stages of their studies. Many appeared to have forgotten the reality of their earlier placements, when they often spent hours preparing each individual activity for a client, or writing and rewriting their client aims. Towards the latter stages of their studies, most of the students attached the highest values to being competent in carrying out what they considered to be very specific tasks such as assessing a stammer, learning sign language or identifying dysphagia. Although some of these skills were clearly tied to a specific client group, many of the students did come to acknowledge the wider applications of their experience during the course of their reflections during the interviews.

> Interacting with people and professionals is something you always need no matter where you are, and I think they have to be the skills that are consistent and that you can use well. I think that's probably the most transferable skill… building relationships with people. **Anya**

Placement allocation…'I thought I would hate it, but now it's where I see my future and I am really excited'

There is no uniform method of allocating placements to students. Most universities strive to provide each student with some paediatric and some adult experience in order to meet the guidelines that suggest students need to work with a range of clients. Students are often asked for their preferences and, within the constraints of the local SLT services, they may secure placements in their preferred contexts. The period of time leading up to students finding out where they are going on placement is often highly charged, both for the students and for academic staff. Many students have very strong ideas about the types of clients that they think they want to work with. These ideas may be formed prior to university as a result of personal or work experience, or they may develop out of lectures that particularly inspire a student. This was certainly the case for many of the students interviewed, but many also revealed just how much they enjoyed placements that they had initially thought they would dislike or find particularly difficult. Keeping an open mind and having a positive attitude towards all placements was one of most common pieces of advice from the students interviewed for this book.

Top tips

All of the students interviewed for this book were asked to offer their 'top five tips' to others who were about to embark on placement with a particular client group. Experienced, practising clinical educators were asked to carry out the same exercise. Interestingly, much of the advice offered by the students was highly transferable to any speech and language therapy context, whereas the advice from clinicians tended to be much more specific to their client group. One reason for this may be that the students are regularly exposed to discussion about transferable skills at university and had all gained experience of working with a range of client groups over the previous few years. In contrast, the speech and language therapists had all been practising in their specialist field for at least two years and consequently were more able to provide specific advice or, alternatively, less able to provide more generic advice. Despite these differences, the advice offered by both groups fell into the same three broad themes: knowledge and practice, working with your clinical educator and attitude. Both the students and clinicians provided many valuable pieces of advice that offer an insight into the experiences of other students and the expectations of clinical educators.

Top transferable tips from students

Working with your clinical educator

- When observing, observe the therapist as well as the client and note the strategies they use.

- Be prepared for any possible emotional impacts of placement and talk to your clinical educator about how you are feeling.

- Accept that it is OK if you don't know everything, but be prepared to find out if you need to.

- Discuss the theory behind what you are doing with your clinical educator. This allows you to demonstrate your competence.

- Ask for lots of feedback from your clinical educator. The positive feedback will build your confidence and the critical feedback will help you develop and improve your skills.

Knowledge and practice

- Spend time prior to placement reading about the conditions that you are most likely to encounter.

- Make an information pack prior to placement that contains all of the key information so that you can refer to this during sessions.

- Dress appropriately and modestly.

- Once on placement, do some reading each day. Try to read books and articles that are related to the clients you are seeing in placement.

- Always consider the functional aspects of therapy and make sure that what you are doing is relevant to each individual client.

- Consider the impact of the communication impairment on your client's everyday life.

- Recognise the importance of being part of a multidisciplinary team. Talk to other professionals about clients to gain a more holistic view and to further your understanding of the role of different professionals.

- Take a flexible and adaptable approach to sessions. Provide steps up and down in session plans but also have further adaptations that you could make in mind.

- Make clear and organised recordings during sessions because this will help when you come to write up case notes after the session.

Attitude

- Always remember that the client is the focus of a session. Try to be yourself and focus on the client, not your own fears. Be responsive to their needs and try not to focus too much on your own performance. Although this is sometimes difficult, it will help you to establish a better relationship with your clients.

- Be organised and pro-active with your learning.

- Be open to enjoying the experience of all placements. Keep an open mind; don't allow yourself to be convinced about the client group that you want to work with in the future because this may have a negative impact on how much you enjoy and learn from other placements.

- Being young does not mean that your opinions won't be respected.

- Show enthusiasm!

Top transferable tips from clinical educators

Working with your clinical educator

- Be prepared to discuss previous placements with your clinical educator in an organised manner. Try not to be just descriptive, but talk about what you have learned from your experiences. Your clinical educator can then take your previous experience into account in terms of the support offered.

- Make your clinical educator aware of any anxieties you may have that you may need some extra support with on placement.

- Discuss personal goals and learning outcomes during the early stages of placement and let your clinical educator know about anything in particular that you would like to see or do so that they have time to try to make arrangements.

- If you are asked to do something that you don't feel competent to do, discuss this with your clinical educator.

Knowledge and practice

- Remember that you have developed skills on other placements that are transferrable to all contexts…case note writing, report writing, taking a case history.

- Take the initiative to do your own research and reading related to what you are seeing on placement. Don't forget to feed this back to your clinical educator.

- Be aware of the role of other professionals and how speech and language therapists fit into the setting.

- Be aware of both formal and informal methods of assessing a client.

- Learn about your client as an individual from as many people as you can.

- Record as much as you can during a session but do not let this detract from your interaction. Having your own proforma and practising recording with this prior to sessions will help. Experiment with different forms of recording (tables, tick boxes) so that you know what works best for you.

- Give clients as much time as they need to respond.

- Develop clear and consistent feedback to give to your client and always bear in mind the purpose of your feedback.

- Be prepared to think flexibly and take an adaptable approach to sessions. Some students feel that they have 'failed' when their session plan needs to be adapted. On the contrary, this flexibility is a great strength.

- Take some work with you so that you can use any time between appointments productively.

Attitude

- Try to enjoy the experience. You are not supposed to know everything so take every opportunity to ask questions and learn. Clinical educators prefer a student who is confident enough to ask questions and is honest about their level of knowledge and understanding.

- Be prepared to have a go at things and show enthusiasm!

4 Children with speech, language and communication impairments

Communication difficulties are one of the most common diagnoses in early childhood and children may present with either delayed or disordered speech and language. A developmental *delay* means that the sequence of speech and language development is typical but behind in terms of the age at which particular aspects are mastered, whereas a *disorder* implies either a significant delay or a pattern of speech and language development which differs from the norm (Stackhouse & Wells, 1997). Children with speech impairments usually make phonemic or phonological errors whereas children with a language impairment present with receptive and/or expressive language difficulties. There are few studies investigating the incidence and prevalence of speech and language impairments in children and the available statistics vary considerably. The incidence of speech and language impairment over the period of one year amongst children without any other co-morbid condition has been estimated at 16.3% (Broomfield & Dodd, 2004), although this only includes those children referred for speech and language therapy and the rates are known to vary across regions. Speech and language therapists are involved both in early intervention and prevention of speech and language disorders, and in the remediation of impairments through the process of assessment and intervention. The services are delivered under a range of guises: individual or group therapy, parent-based or child-centred therapy, and are delivered across a variety of settings. Clients also range in age from preschool through to secondary school age.

Ten students looked back at their paediatric placements, discussing the way in which services were delivered and the types of assessment and therapy that they were engaged in during their time on placement. Many had limited experience working with children and their parents, and the students reflected on these new challenges and the insights that they gained.

Setting

The variety experienced by students on paediatric placements illustrates the wide range of settings in which speech and language therapists work with children. Some of the students were based in a community clinic and the children attended for appointments with a parent or guardian. Others travelled between different schools in an area to work with children, and some of the students were based at a specialist language unit attached to a particular school. In fact, many of the students saw their clients in a variety of these settings within a single placement.

Alyson was based in a community clinic, though she spent much of her time travelling to local schools to see her clients if they did not attend their appointments at the clinic.

> It was a clinic based service, however not many children came into the service…they got a lot of DNAs, [did not attend] people did not really turn up. So a lot of their service was going into mainstream schools and nurseries, and targeting the children in that way. We went to local primary schools and nurseries attached to schools. We saw a range of children with different communication needs within the community. **Alyson**

Amira had a similar experience, working with preschool and primary school-aged children both in the community centre and in nurseries and mainstream schools. She also worked alongside her CE to run regular 'drop-in' sessions for parents and children who had been referred to speech and language therapy by their health visitors. Matt spent half of his placement within a language unit for children with a diagnosis of specific language impairment (SLI). The other days were spent in a range of services seeing children with a variety of speech, language and communication needs (SLCN).

> I did a couple of community clinics, so that's [children] from age two up…I did initial assessments there. And I went into mainstream primary schools, either for assessments or discussion with the teachers. **Matt**

Working in schools

Many of the students worked with children and education staff within the school environment. Molly worked with children who had SLI, joining a team of SLTs who provided outreach services to children at the different schools that Molly and her CE visited regularly.

> I would meet my CE in a health centre and have that as the base, then just go out from there. I was [working with children who had] SLI in mainstream school, both high school and primary school...they were all different schools, going to each pupil at whatever school they went to, and they [the children] would have an hour out of their day. The majority of the day was spent in the schools. [We would] have lunch in the clinic and then get back about 3.30 to do case notes. So [I would] get in at 8.30 and then leave at 4.30. **Molly**

Alyson saw some of her clients in a clinic setting, and others at the school they attended. However, she preferred working in schools because she felt that the children were more relaxed and so able to engage more easily with sessions.

> I probably feel most at home in the school environment. They are natural places for the children...you're taking them out of their classroom, but they still feel quite at home because you're working in their library or you're working in a room where they do their phonics group. It's not such an alien environment, so the children I think always feel a bit more at ease. **Alyson**

Several of the students experienced working within a language unit during the course of their placement. In recent years, there has been a sharp rise in the number of language units in the UK. Most units are attached to mainstream schools so that the children are able to integrate with their peers, and spend some time each week in mainstream classes in many cases. The majority of their education, however, takes place within these language-based classrooms and is facilitated by a range of specialist staff. Although there are no set national guidelines, most language units have similar criteria in order for a child to gain a place within this specialist setting. Botting, Crutchley and Conti-Ramsden (1998) refer to four common criteria: the child has a statement of special educational needs (SEN); the child has age-appropriate nonverbal cognitive skills; the child's primary difficulty is with language; and, finally, that the child would benefit from a structured setting with a small number of peers. Martina was based full-time at a language unit attached to a school, which catered for 18 local children with SLI.

> They were there full time for a minimum of two terms, but because their language needs were so severe, some of them were there for reception, year 1 and year 2, so it was a Key Stage 1[1] language base. It was attached to a school, but it was a classroom in its own right. It was in the Key Stage 1 area of the school and the children did integrate with the rest of the school. So there was a different teaching structure that went on and obviously the teacher was specially trained in special educational needs, language, that kind of thing. There was a high level of teaching assistant support and there was also a speech and language therapist on site. I worked quite closely with the learning support assistants so I could see the children in the classroom. **Martina**

All of the students enjoyed working in the school setting, though it was not without its challenges. Martina found that, despite being in a specialist language unit, the environment presented challenges for both herself and her client because the sessions took place in the corner of a busy classroom within the unit rather than a separate therapy room.

> I was doing an activity with a boy and we were practising /s/ clusters. He was a really quiet boy and I was really struggling to hear…sometimes I actually missed whether he did the /s/ cluster or not because of the general noise of the classroom. I know when you're a teacher or when you work in that environment, you get used to zoning out the noise, but that was a challenge…the noise and distraction…a distraction for me, but also a distraction for the children. **Martina**

---

1 The HM Government (2002) *Education Act* defines Key Stage 1 as 'the period beginning at the same time as the school year in which he attains the age of six and ending at the same time as the school year in which the majority of pupils in his class attain the age of seven.'

Matt worked in a number of different schools during the course of his placement. Although some students found this challenging, Matt felt that he benefitted by gaining an insight into the education setting that he would not have gained were he based only in one school.

> It was nice speaking to different teachers…seeing how different schools are [from each] other was really interesting as well. Depending on how they are run, our role as a speech therapist can be viewed very, very differently and that was one of the things that tended to crop up a lot. You assume at first when you go to placement that all the schools are the same. Some schools know exactly what they are doing, and then some other schools need loads of support and that was one of the things that surprised me. A lot of the schools didn't have many children with speech and language difficulties, so when a child did crop up, they panicked a lot more. Whereas some schools, there would be a lot more children with speech and language difficulties, but the teachers were able to take it more in their stride, and had a lot more resources to be able to deal with that. **Matt**

Most of the students gained experience of working closely with other professionals, often forming very close working relationships with teaching assistants and special educational needs coordinators (SENCOs), who coordinate support for children with special educational needs (SEN). They also liaise between the school, parents and external services such as educational psychology and speech and language therapy. Many of the students also liaised with educational psychologists, although this was usually to share information and refer clients as opposed to regular meetings.

> The multidisciplinary side of it was definitely interesting. [There were] a lot of educational psychologists involved, we were waiting for their reports to come through to be able to analyse the data. I had to ring a couple of times to ask their opinion…they'd seen the child within the last week so what were the results of the assessment or could they send the report. Sometimes we were just chasing up to see if they felt they needed to be involved. **Alyson**

In the primary and secondary schools, the students reported that they had very little interaction with class teachers because the children came out of their classroom to have speech and language therapy sessions in a separate room. In these cases, the students liaised with the SENCO and teaching assistants whereas the students on placement within a nursery school setting tended to work more directly with the class teachers.

> In nursery I delivered a care plan to a teacher...I did informal assessment first and then based on that assessment, I wrote a care plan. From the informal assessment I found that she [the child] was expressively and receptively delayed, so it was working on naming, doing 'Derbyshire type'[2] things, and I gave some materials as well to go with it and demonstrated that to her. **Amira**

The students based in one school found that they were able to build up close working relationships with staff and enjoyed the fact that they began to feel like part of the team within the school. Although largely a positive experience, some of the students did experience difficult situations, usually as a result of lack of understanding of each other's roles within the school.

> In one school which I remember going to...it was completely different to any of the other schools and that was a bit of a shock...as a student you're just sat there and you don't know what to do and the speech therapist was trying to explain what our role was in the school, and the SENCO had completely the wrong idea of it. The Trust was rolling out some new assessments that the school could do on all the children in nursery and reception that might highlight difficulties. The speech therapist was suggesting, "Well maybe you might do this assessment on some of the children"...the SENCO was just like, "No, why would I want to do that?" It was getting across to her that just because you can't see any difficulties...a lot of [people] think of speech, they forget language and they say the speech is fine. And it's not just the speech, you've got to think "Do they [the children] understand you?" **Matt**

---

2 Knowles, W. & Masidlover, M. (1982) *The Derbyshire Language Scheme.* Derbyshire County Council

Despite occasional difficulties such as these, the students worked hard to form relationships with staff and found that teaching assistants in particular played a vitally important role within the classroom. Many of the students found that teaching assistants knew the clients very well and so could provide more information about how they were functioning in the classroom.

> There are ways of going about telling a TA how to do something and respecting the TA's position…respecting that they know the child better than you do and they're carrying over that work every week. Involve the TAs in the sessions, so if we were playing a game I'd do it with three of us, the child, me and the TA. Then they'd do that during the week, so they already knew a bit about what to do… It depended on the TA…how much they were willing to take on board, but the ones we had were pretty good. **Molly**

Martina also worked closely with the classroom staff because many carried out the therapy that she had designed for the children following assessment. She found that sharing their knowledge of the children helped all of the team to gain a deeper understanding of how each child was functioning so that tailored support could be offered.

> We did a lot of feeding back to teaching assistants because they were the ones who carried out sessions and worked one-to-one with the children. On a couple of the activities we asked the TAs to come and sit in with us to see the kind of things that we were doing. [We discussed] the strengths that the children had and areas of need, so that when they were in the classroom, they were able to model the kind of things that we were doing and support the child. I had a good chat with the teacher of the class about one child because there were certain things he was struggling with. I talked about giving him some visual vocabulary to support a story, writing activities and teaching the vocabulary…we had a few lengthy conversations about that. These were complex children, so sometimes we didn't all know the answers, and by working together it helped us understand the child better…it was good experience to talk to the teachers…we had a nice rapport come the end. **Martina**

Working in a community clinic

The majority of the students spent at least part of their placement in a community paediatric clinic. Most of the children had been referred into the service by their nursery or primary school for an initial assessment. Seeing children in the clinic setting allowed the students to gain information from parents and also to model interaction skills or therapy techniques that parents could implement in the home environment.

> I was based in a clinic, so children came into clinic and we'd see them there, all ages really. We'd have perhaps two initials [appointments] in the day, perhaps one therapy session and one review [of a client]. There were two children a week that I saw regularly so I was able to plan my sessions for them. They booked in all the children in the morning, and then the afternoon slot would be notes and reports. One thing that I found difficult was there seemed to be a lot of failing to attend sessions. **David**

Poor attendance was an issue that all of the students in the community paediatric setting experienced.

> It was difficult because I felt sometimes I'd prepare for a session and spend quite a lot of time on a session and sometimes I didn't get to show what I had to give. The DNAs were quite difficult because they obviously did not consistently receive speech therapy and they forgot what they'd learnt…so that makes you almost fall back instead of progress. **Donna**

As a result of non-attendance, some of the students found that they had significant periods of free time during their days, which they filled by looking at unfamiliar assessments and doing extra reading related to their clients. Others were able to discuss their planned sessions with their clinical educator and gain feedback. Some found that working in a clinic with only their clinical educator for support could be difficult in terms of learning about the wider picture of how speech and language difficulties affect a child and their family. The students who split their time between a community clinic and educational settings felt as though they gained a deeper insight into their clients as a result of observing them in a range of settings.

I was doing paediatric community clinic work, so that was mainly preschool and primary school age range really... going to nursery, doing primary school visits. It was a community clinic so we were getting referrals and parents were bringing children in, but as part of that we'd then follow up going doing a preschool visit after. **Lara**

Working with children

Whilst some students had previous experience of being around and interacting with young children, for many this was their first time and they found this one of the most daunting aspects of their placement.

I'd not really worked with children before, so I felt like I didn't know how they'd react. One of my goals was to manage different behaviours because I wasn't really sure how the children would be with me. I worked really well with them, so it wasn't as challenging [as I had expected]. I had one child who I did continuous work with every week and eventually I was allowed to just run all those sessions. And he had really poor attention, but I'd use my imagination to get good therapy...using different visual things, and a lot of games. **Amira**

Some had concerns around what they would talk to the children about, whereas others were worried about balancing their role in engaging the child whilst maintaining their professional role in sessions that were observed by their clinical educator. Despite these concerns, all of the students felt that this was an area where their skills and confidence improved dramatically over the course of their placement and it ceased to be an issue after the initial few weeks.

As a student, I'm not used to being around children, so that was one thing for me to learn, just how to interact with children. I feel comfortable with it now, but I remember at first feeling really silly having to act silly...and you've got your clinical educator watching you and that was always something that I was worried about. But I knew that would probably come with experience, that I would

> feel more comfortable with children. I think that was my main apprehension before placement. I feel fine now…for example, I said to one child, "What have you been doing in class today?" and he said, "I'm not telling you." I think at first if a kid had said that to me, I would have gone "er, OK" but I just said, "Right, OK, well I'll guess"…so I started just guessing really silly things and getting that rapport with a child that I never would have had a few weeks ago. If they're not watching you (the CE), you kind of you don't care if you say something silly because it's only the child. But you wouldn't want to be as silly in front of an adult, so it's just getting used to that. **Matt**

Many of the students commented on the variability of the quality of interactions achieved during a session. Sometimes this was due to the inherent unpredictability of children in terms of their mood, engagement and behaviour, all of which impacted on the success of a session. The quality of interaction also depended on the student and their own developing skills.

> Some of the feedback I got was "You're really confident some days and then other days you're a bit more reluctant and a bit less confident to do things". But I think that's quite a natural thing. **Anya**

Donna found that following the child's lead was often the most effective way to achieve the session aims because the child engaged more readily. A flexible approach was highlighted by many of the students as the most important strategy for a successful session with their client.

> Accept that you often need to go with the flow rather than being structured. Also accept that sometimes your session isn't going to go to plan, and that might be because of you or or just the way the child's feeling, because obviously the child's quite nervous coming into a clinic with a stranger trying to get him to say words. I'd just say follow his lead really, and through play, they're almost fooled into being assessed. **Donna**

Alyson was also keen to share her advice about keeping children motivated throughout sessions. She found that each child was responsive to different rewards and games, and so spending time getting to know the clients and gaining this information from parents or guardians and classroom staff was crucial. She also soon learned that each child needed a range of games and toys to stay engaged, and that bringing out materials that worked well in one session did not guarantee that they would have the same impact in the subsequent session with the same child.

> We actually had one child…at the end of the session we'd play a reward game, and he kept asking for this particular game we'd never heard of. My CE actually went and bought it and this kid was just so responsive to it, and we got more expressive data out of him than we'd ever got before. So I think just being aware of what the child wants to do as much as anything, not just assuming that if one game works for that child it's going to work for the next four you see on the same day. **Alyson**

Despite his initial reservations and apprehensions about working with children, Matt had a very positive experience on placement, and this was largely due to him getting to know the children as individuals.

> I liked it more than I thought I would…I was always quite set that I'll probably work with adults, but after working in paediatrics, I really did enjoy it and once you get the rapport with the children it's really nice to see their personalities coming out. **Matt**

Caseload

Most of the students had a varied caseload, consisting of clients with a range of speech and language delays and disorders. The children varied widely in age, from preschool through to secondary school age. Primary school-aged children made up the majority of the students' caseloads and referrals into the service predominantly came from parents or class teachers.

> Generally it was a lot of [children with] developmental delay where they were a few months behind but the parents were really worried…or the preschool were saying "Their

> speech isn't clear and all of their peers' speech is really clear". **Lara**

The students who worked with preschool children tended to experience a wider range of impairments because some children were yet to be diagnosed with particular conditions and so came under the remit of a general paediatric caseload.

> We had [children with] phonological delay and disorder, we had one who had juvenile arthritis that was affecting her jaw and therefore her articulation. We had some quite severe, quite complex children, with learning difficulties but [they were] in the process of being diagnosed as to what the real breakdown was. They were querying autistic spectrum disorder for one boy but what we saw wasn't really fitting when we were actually assessing…we were thinking, "Are we just trying to put him in a box?" **Alyson**

Despite the students being based in mainstream settings, many did work with clients who had recognised medical conditions, or were in the process of diagnosis if they were seen in a preschool setting.

> Surprisingly, some of the youngest children I saw were actually 18 months…referred by health visitors. For that particular child it was tongue tie and the parents were worried that it was going to affect his speech in later life, which was a very surprising client I didn't expect to see. The other ones had grommets, quite often they were 2 to 3 [years old], with delayed language and speech. But they were just the surprising ones, the other ones were your typical language and phonology delay. **Donna**

Like Donna, most of the students had anticipated a relatively predictable caseload. Many were surprised at the complexity of their clients and identified a number of factors that made working with their clients more challenging than they had anticipated. They found that the interaction between the different domains of speech and language often created a complex picture; many of the children presented with multi-faceted speech and language impairments that included phonology, syntax, semantic and pragmatic issues and it could be difficult to tease these apart. The range in severity of the speech and language impairments that the children presented with was also unexpected for many of the students. Vanessa described her initial session with an 11-year old child that she saw in a mainstream secondary school.

> She was just so unresponsive. I've never seen a child like that really. We did the ACE[3], she got the first centile in absolutely everything…clearly she had cognitive issues. We did the picture naming. She got every single one wrong, but after the fifth picture she just wouldn't even respond because she didn't know, but she wouldn't say she didn't know either. She would just sit there and stare at the picture. I felt so sorry for her, because I thought "how's she got through school, she obviously doesn't have a clue what's going on in the day." It was awful, actually. I wonder how she got through school without any extra support. **Vanessa**

Conversely, some of the students felt that they worked with a less diverse range of clients than they had expected and found that this was one of the less enjoyable aspects of their placement.

> I think the oldest that I saw was perhaps about 10 [years old]. It was mainly speech sounds and language as the main caseload. I didn't expect to be seeing the same types of clients the whole time, there was a lot of repetition and there didn't seem to be a lot of variety of different things we'd be seeing. Because it was community, I thought it'd be a mixture of things we'd be seeing, but it just seemed quite repetitive. **David**

These reflections show that even working with the same client group in comparable environments can lead to different experiences for students depending on the particular service and location that they are placed.

Although none of the students felt that their placements were particularly emotionally demanding, many did feel a great deal of empathy for their clients and their families. Working with a range of clients helped the students to understand the impacts that speech and language impairments can have on a child's self-esteem and relationships.

---

3 Adams, C., Cooke, R., Crutchley, A., Hesketh, A., & Reeves, D. (2001). *Assessment of Comprehension and Expression 6-11 (ACE)*. London: GL Assessment.

> There was a child in the group, he had quite a severe phonological disorder and he'd only been seen for a brief assessment so we didn't know very much about him and mum usually brought him. Mum could understand him so well but he was literally unintelligible. One week [his] nan came in and clearly couldn't understand him and he was so distressed. She was talking about lunch and he was saying something none of us could understand and I thought it must be so annoying for him, in his head he's saying it perfectly clearly. **Vanessa**

Working with bilingual children

Research shows that over half of all paediatric speech and language therapists in England work with bilingual children (Winter, 1999). There is strong evidence to suggest that, far from being a cause of any difficulties, bilingualism is often an advantage in terms of speech and language development (Cummins, 2000; Royal College of Speech and Language Therapists, 2007). However, this does not mean that children are able to easily acquire a second language, nor does it preclude them from developing speech and language impairments. Several of the students worked with bilingual children, though they all worked in English and did not access an interpreter. Martina worked with a 7-year-old child and described the challenges involved in diagnosing his difficulties.

> He was right at the beginning of his time at the school and he had some social and pragmatic issues. We didn't really come to a conclusion about him in the weeks that we were there, because it wasn't long enough. He needed a lot of time to settle into a new environment and to have more assessments done, because we were all quite puzzled. We didn't have any interpreters. He did have a few English words. What he used to do, when you asked him point to the bird before you point to the cat, he would then repeat that back to you. He didn't understand that he was supposed to carry out a task, just echolalia. **Martina**

The current recommendations are for the child to receive therapy in the languages that they are most frequently exposed to (Royal College of Speech and Language Therapists, 2007), though some families opt for their child to receive therapy in English, even if this is not the main language spoken at home, because they feel this be more beneficial in terms of their child's education. This situation was something that Martina experienced with another bilingual child on her placement in the language unit.

> One of them had been there [at the language unit] for a couple of years. He came into the school, with no language, neither his own family language nor English. And because he was taking such a long time to develop language, the family decided it would be better for him to learn just English because this is where they were staying. And against the advice of the professionals, they decided for him to speak English. He had started to talk in sentences, he had developed a lot. **Martina**

Vanessa also had a number of bilingual children on her caseload, and found that she needed to take an extended language history from the child's family to gain a sense of the language environment that the child was exposed to both in terms of immediate family and extended family. She worked regularly with one bilingual child in group sessions who had selective mutism. The prevalence of selective mutism is higher in immigrant language minority children, though it can be difficult to diagnose due to the fact that these children may simply have limited skills in the new language being acquired (Toppelberg, Tabors, Coggins, Lum, & Burger, 2005).

> She never spoke and she had such a blank facial expression. And mum was, like, "She does talk, she does talk at home loads" and mum recorded her speaking at home and showed it us. One week I was running a little late and I heard this little voice behind me, and it was this little girl, she was chatting away to her mum. The minute she saw me she went quiet. So that was interesting, that's quite common in the bilingual population. **Vanessa**

Working with parents and taking case histories

Most of the students worked with the parents or guardians of their clients during the course of their placements. Preschool children or children who were seen in a community clinic were usually accompanied by their parents and the students were involved in taking case histories, providing advice and giving feedback to parents. Some of the students also worked in a more direct way with parents, helping to run group sessions that encouraged parents to develop their own interaction skills. The prospect of working with parents in this context was daunting for most of the students, and in many cases they were more nervous about these interactions than about their direct work with the children.

Taking a case history

Taking a case history was something that most of the students had experienced during previous placements. This helped some to feel more confident about this aspect of interacting with their clients' parents, whereas others continued to find it a challenge.

> I felt quite confident. I'd done case histories before, and I read the file beforehand, you're kind of prepared, and I wasn't on my own ever in the room, my clinical educator was always there. So actually I thought if she [the client's mother] says something and I don't pick up on it, my clinical educator will make a note and at the end she'll come back to it, or she'll step in. I was happy that there was someone there but she didn't feel the need to step in at any point. There were one or two [occasions] when she just clarified a few points. I think I was able to get the bulk of the information and I made sure I had a proforma to start with so I knew what areas I was going to question and work through, so it flowed a bit easier than just plucking questions out of the air and hoping for the best. **Alyson**

One of the aspects that students found most difficult was to observe and interact with the child whilst simultaneously speaking to their parents to gain information. Managing these sessions was often a challenge, and there was great variation in the response from parents to the case history questions. Some parents were keen to provide lots of detailed information whereas others were more reluctant, and the students felt as though they needed to prompt much more to gain information about the background of a child.

> You're trying to find out as much as you can from parents, and it's hard if they're not quite as responsive as others. I found it quite difficult doing case histories. I was a little bit unsure and I was trying to ask the questions and write notes at the same time, scribble things down as fast as I could and it didn't seem [like] a natural conversation, it just seemed a bit, maybe, awkward at times. You have a case history form to fill out, but often you can't follow the set questions that are there because some aren't appropriate, some you need to ask further additional questions. **David**

Despite these initial challenges, many of the students felt their skills developed over time and found their own solutions that helped them to manage particularly difficult sessions. Being open and honest with the parents and explaining the reasons for asking particular questions appeared to create a more relaxed environment in which many of the parents were more forthcoming with information.

> I think being able to explain why you're asking questions, that was the biggest thing for me. When I'm asking for a case history, saying, "Some of these questions seem really silly and I do apologise in advance but as I go along I'll try and explain why I'm asking them. I'm not being nosey I just want to get a clear picture of how your child's doing at the moment." I think parents really appreciate that honesty and parents often go, "Oh, OK, that makes sense." I don't think you should ever get to a stage where you're condescending and 'I know best', because, ultimately, parents are the expert on their own child. **Lara**

Feeding back to parents

At the end of an assessment or therapy session, many of the students were required to provide feedback about the child to their parents, giving an immediate evaluation of the session whilst presenting the information in a sensitive and accessible way. For many of the students, this was the most anxiety-provoking aspect of a paediatric placement. As their knowledge and experience grew, the process of giving feedback began to come more naturally and the students also gained from observing their clinical educators interacting with parents.

> It was a lot of advice, suggestions for learning early language…I did find it difficult at first. I think I was perhaps [making] it too complex…I think I had to make it quite simple. I observed the person I was working with and saw how she did it, and it made perfect sense and it was a lot easier then. In the end I felt a lot more confident. **David**

The younger students were particularly daunted by the prospect of feeding back to parents because they felt that their advice might not be taken on board due to their age and perceived inexperience. Most found that building strategies for giving feedback into their session plans helped them to feel less nervous and more prepared for these situations.

> I have found it hard with feeding back to parents, because I thought they'd probably look at me [and think], "Oh, she's 20, no kids, who are you to tell me how to look after mine?" I found that more with the younger children that were slow to talk, because you're doing all the modelling and the naming and they probably thought, "I already do that so why are you telling me?" I tried to build it into my session plan, so that I was quite organised. So generally I tried to have a little chat at the beginning to talk things through…then if it was a session where I was giving parents techniques to do, I'd play with the children and then just talk about what I was doing while I was doing it. So [I wasn't] directly saying, "Right, you need to do this, this and this." **Molly**

Vanessa also found that including ideas for feedback in her session plan helped her to feel more prepared and able to offer quality feedback to parents. She practised different ways of phrasing her feedback so that she could find the most clear and sensitive ways to give information to parents and felt that this reduced the demands of carrying out the sessions to some extent.

> That's been one of the most scary things to do. I decided if I did a really structured session plan and a recording with it, I thought that would help my feedback [to parents].

Because gathering your thoughts, thinking of how to say it in an appropriate way and then saying it, is quite a lot to think about when you're a student. So when I went in with that plan I found it so much better. That's more nerve wracking than being with the children, speaking to the parents. They're waiting on every word that you're going to say and they really want you to say something really positive. Sometimes you've got to say not so positive things in a nice way, it's hard. **Vanessa**

Parents' attitudes towards speech and language therapy

The students talked at length about the range of reactions from parents about their child's referral for speech and language therapy assessment.

[There was] a lot of talking to parents and being able to say "Actually we're not that worried and this is the advice"… giving them some strategies and stuff to work on at home. But obviously you are going to have parents that come in thinking "The preschool have referred them but I don't think there's anything wrong", then they find out actually, there's a lot going on with their child and you slowly let them know a bit at a time…explaining to them what's presenting and positive things as well as negative, just so that they're not completely overwhelmed. I think that was the biggest thing I saw on this placement, the way that different parents reacted. **Lara**

The discrepancies between how parents dealt with their child's referral were often linked to who had made that referral to the service. In many cases, the children were referred by health visitors, nursery staff or teachers and the parents who brought their child to the initial session did not have any concerns about their child's speech and language development.

There was a question in the case history which was "How concerned are you about your child's speech and language?", and quite a lot of them weren't concerned at all. And obviously for a child to make progress, there needs to be a lot of support from parents at home and quite often it wasn't the case. I had to explain how important it was. And try and provide them with some sort of homework that was accessible for them to use. Whether they actually did something about it, I'm not quite sure. We had an assessment, we identified there was quite a large level of need, we explained to the parents about that, but following that, they [sometimes] didn't attend, so that was very difficult. **Donna**

Of course, in many cases, parents were extremely worried about their child's speech and language development, and these sessions were often equally challenging for the students.

There were a couple of times in community clinic with some parents who were very concerned about their children understandably. There was one lady whose older son had quite severe autism, and she was concerned about her [younger] son who she'd brought into clinic. That's when you put yourself in the parent's shoes…, you forget that sometimes. I remember being at an annual review for one of the children and the mum and dad were there, and it was a really heated discussion where I felt really uncomfortable. Dad felt that his child's literacy difficulties were because he [the child] was having so much speech therapy in the language unit and speech therapy was the reason he was very disorganised in his narrative and his reading and spelling were poor. There was a lot of emotion from dad and I'd hate to have been in the speech therapist's shoes in that moment, because he was basically blaming her for his son's literacy difficulties and felt that we were saying his son was stupid. But obviously with being in the language unit it wasn't his intelligence or his IQ or cognitive abilities…if I was in that position, I don't know what I'd do. **Matt**

These situations demonstrate the importance of understanding the wider context of the impacts of speech and language difficulties and recognising the range of situations that the children are experiencing both at home and in education. The students all felt supported by their clinical educator and were often able to deal with difficult situations independently.

> There was a child in the group and his mum was extremely anxious, she was leaning over constantly, shouting at him to say it right. And we weren't focusing on output anyway, because it was phonological awareness, so it was just us giving them input. His mum was very anxious…that can impact on the child, they pick up on that, clearly he was. The clinical educator said, "You controlled it really well actually". I didn't actually say anything directly to her, I just moved the child away from that, so gave him something else to think about. You don't want to say "Stop doing it", because you know they're anxious and you can imagine you want your child to be saying exactly everything right. And I think it's good that she wanted to help.   **Vanessa**

Anya attended a number of child protection meetings during the course of her placement. The multidisciplinary team involved in each child's health and welfare would meet with the child's parents and the child would also attend, depending on their age. The meetings varied enormously depending on those involved, but the main focus was on the parents' level of engagement with the services being provided for their child. Anya was able to work with her CE in preparation for these meetings and contribute her own findings about the particular children. Although she did not play an active role during the meetings, she felt as though she gained a great deal from from observing the process.

> It was very different depending on the family backgrounds. With one it was a really positive role, saying the mum's really engaged with the service and the child has come on leaps and bounds. With another, the mum wasn't engaged with the service but the child had got the capacity to become age appropriate within normal limits. So it was about the engagement with the service by the parent, and how the child was doing from a speech and language point of view. It was a lot smaller role than a lot of the other professionals who were there, but I think everyone was interested to know [about the child's speech and language development].   **Anya**

Assessment

Assessment formed a significant part of the students' work with their clients and presented a number of challenges. Maintaining a child's attention, dealing with large amounts of data and learning how to use standardised assessments were the key issues for many of the students. Assessing young children proved particularly challenging due to their short attention span, and the students found that taking a flexible approach integrated with play often helped them to gain the information needed. Alyson found that carrying out frequent, 20-minute sessions worked better for her young clients than one longer session during which the child lost interest. Taking a more flexible approach was also a strategy that Donna adopted following her initial experiences with a preschool child.

> I did standardised assessments such as the Derbyshire Language Scheme[4]. I realised that children were often not very compliant with those sort of things. So you had to follow their lead and take part in a playful activity. So you were almost concealing the fact that you were assessing them. At the beginning for my first assessment with a 3-year-old, I sat down and I made a really, really structured session plan and thought it was great. I got into the session and I didn't follow it at all, because the child just didn't want to do it. They wanted to do their own thing. And I found that being flexible actually elicited more expressive language from them. I just had to have some goals and I made sure that I achieved those goals. And sometimes even then that wasn't possible because of the child's attention and listening so it might have taken two sessions. **Donna**

Some of the students found that they were able to use informal approaches to assessment where appropriate and their departments often had their own screens that the students used.

> In the [community] clinic it was the departmental screen, so it would be the informal one that we used there. There was [one for] young children, which was word levels, and then the older child one was more high level

---

4   Knowles, W. & Masidlover, M. (1982). *The Derbyshire Language Scheme*. Derbyshire County Council.

language. In the mainstream schools it was just formal assessments. **Matt**

Some of the students had experience of working with children on earlier placements, whereas for others this was their first time despite being in their final year of study. Becoming familiar with a wide range of standardised assessments was particularly challenging for those students who were unfamiliar with this client group, but they all felt that this was an area in which their skills had really developed by the end of their placements.

> I did a CELF[5], the BPVS[6], the STAP[7], the TALC[8] for the social use of language. I didn't have lots of experience with using lots of formal assessments and I did struggle. For instance, with the CELF, I needed to do every subsection and they're all presented differently, you ask them in a different way, sometimes you repeat or you don't. So getting used to all of the different subsections and how you present them, and then scoring them…It was brilliant because I now know how to do that, but I didn't to begin with and so I did struggle. And the whole process of going to the right section to get the standard score, the raw score, age equivalent…it's a process that takes a lot of getting used to. I think when I'm in a job and I've done that ten times, I'm going to be as quick as the next person but when you don't know the whole process, it's a tricky process. And when they give you a response that you're not expecting, or you have to transcribe their response and it's very unintelligible. And when you're online doing it and you're being watched by someone else, the whole process becomes quite stifled. But I'm pleased to say that I definitely developed in that area. **Martina**

---

5   Semmel, E., Wiig, E.H., & Secord, W. (2006b). *Clinical Evaluation of Language Fundamentals-4 (CELF4)*. London: Pearson Assessment.

6   Dunn, L.M., Dunn, D.M., Sewell, J., Styles, B., Bryzyska, B., Shamson, Y. et al. (2009). *British Picture Vocabulary Scales-3 (BPVS-3)*. London: GL Assessment Limited.

7   Armstrong, S. & Ainley, M. (2012). *South Tyneside Assessment of Phonology 2 (STAP)*. St Mabyn, UK: STASS Publications.

8   Elks, L. & McLachlan, H. (2007). *Test of Abstract Language Comprehension (TALC)*. St Mabyn, UK: STASS Publications.

Alyson also found that formal assessment could be time-consuming. Once the assessment scores had been converted into percentiles or age equivalents, the challenge then lay in interpreting the information to guide further assessment or therapy.

> I think that was the biggest challenge, just having all this data and being, like, "What does it really mean?" and having to break it down and not necessarily always having the time needed, you've got so many children you've got to see. **Alyson**

The students discussed a number of ways in which they dealt with these challenges. Many sought support and guidance from their clinical educator, particularly during the early stages of their placement when they felt that they had less knowledge and confidence about administering formal assessments.

> I used the pre-school CELF[9] and I did hundreds of STAPs… At first she'd do it with me, I'd have my own copy and then eventually I could just do it on my own. You have to be quick with transcription, but it's a lot easier once you've done it loads of times. And I used other ones like the CLEAR[10] and the DEAP[11]. I found the CLEAR really easy to do. **Amira**

Alyson initially found having her sessions observed by her clinical educator to be a daunting prospect, particularly when she was carrying out standardised assessments. However, she soon found that her CE was extremely supportive and allowed Alyson to carry out the assessments independently, only stepping in occasionally to guide her and model ways to elicit responses from some of the children. Practising autonomously with the support of her CE helped Alyson to grow in confidence and she was also able to spend some time researching the range of paediatric speech and language assessments that were available, which she felt helped to further increase her knowledge and skills.

---

9 Semmel, E., Wiig, E.H., & Secord, W. (2006a). *CELF Pre-school 2 UK (Clinical Evaulation of Language Fundamentals)*. London, UK: Pearson Assessment.

10 Keeling, M. & Keeling, K. (2006). *CLEAR: Phonology Screening Assessment*. Splisby: CLEAR Resources.

11 Dodd, B., Hua, Z., Crosbie, S., Holm, A., & Ozanne, A. (2006). *Diagnostic Evaluation of Articulation and Phonology (DEAP)*. London, UK: Pearson Assessment.

> Being aware of what assessments are out there, I think that's where I lacked quite a lot of knowledge. I'd had paediatric placements and you find in clinics they have set assessments that they do. So I knew the ones that I'd done on another placement but this clinic had a lot of assessments that I'd never heard of. I think that actually maybe having a bit more knowledge of what they at least tested [would have been useful], even if I didn't know how to carry them out, but being able to say, "OK, we need to do some verb comprehension so we're going to get this out". **Alyson**

Many of the students talked about their confidence growing over the course of their placement, particularly in relation to carrying out formal assessments that require a specific procedure. For many, their confidence grew as their skills improved and this was often simply down to practise and experience.

> We did assessment at least twice a day…the STAP and the CELF were the main standardised ones we did. It was quite repetitive, but it was good practice, I think it was a good thing actually. When I started the placement, I hadn't got much confidence and lacked a few skills. It was one thing that was mentioned at the end [of placement], I had gained a lot more skills in carrying out the assessments, she saw my progression throughout the placement. **David**

Therapy

Despite all of the students being in the final year of their degree, some had previously carried out only assessment with children, and these placements provided their first opportunity to plan and deliver therapy. Their experiences illustrate the range of ways in which intervention can be delivered. Most of the students delivered a combination of direct individual therapy and group sessions, and many also provided training and advice to parents and educational staff. The type of intervention offered depended on a range of factors: the age of the child, parental preferences and service policy.

Individual therapy

Most of the students saw at least one client regularly for individual direct therapy sessions. This was one of the most positive aspects of placement for many of the students, who felt that they learned a great deal and were able to put many of their developing skills into practice.

> I enjoyed it more than I expected. Whenever I've been in clinics, I've not really enjoyed language work, but I enjoyed working with the SLI kids. Maybe it's that I saw them every week for an hour…maybe it's because it was more intense. I was making relationships with the kids. I really enjoyed working with the SLI clients. The ones that we were working with were all doing narration or Colourful Semantics.[12] They had sentence strips to help them form longer sentences… subject, verb, object, location. **Molly**

Those who worked directly with their clients reflected on the individual differences between the children. Although this is something that had been discussed within lectures, the students felt that this direct experience really helped them to understand the heterogeneous nature of a paediatric caseload and to tailor their interaction style and intervention approaches accordingly.

> There was a boy that was 3, we were working on his speech. He was really tuned in and his speech was literally the only problem, his language ability was brilliant, his attention and listening were fabulous, and you forgot he was only 3. But for another 3-year-old I saw, there was no way it would have been appropriate to do direct therapy. I think that can only be learned with experience. I don't think you can say there's a definitive answer…some children at 6 are not ready for therapy. That was really good experience. **Leah**

Some of the students were able to work with their clients throughout the whole of their client's time with the speech and language therapy service; from initial assessment to discharge. This was one of the most rewarding aspects

---

12   Bryan, A. (1997) Colourful semantics: Thematic role therapy. In S. Chiat, J. Law and J. Marshall (Eds), *Language Disorders in Children and Adults: Psycholinguistic approaches to therapy*. London: Whurr.

and the students gained a great deal of satisfaction from being a part of the entire journey.

> A lot of them I saw all the way through and we discharged them in my last week. It was mainly because they achieved their long-term aims and that they had enough support either in school or within nursery or at home. So a particular child was getting brilliant input at home and at nursery, and we'd given him an 8-week block and actually he had grown so much. He was self-monitoring and you could just tell he was going to keep progressing. **Alyson**

Leah took on a more consultative role, training nursery staff and teaching assistants to deliver packages of therapy. All of the students felt that this approach could be beneficial to both the children and the service because it allowed the speech and language therapists to work directly with those children who would benefit most, whilst ensuring that all of the children on the caseload received appropriate input.

> With some of the older children, say they needed three or four word level input or word-finding things, they had packs all made up so that the assistant could just pick up a pack and then they'd do it in the language unit, it was really efficient. **Vanessa**

Group therapy

Group therapy was a common way to deliver intervention, and something that most of the students grew to enjoy despite initially feeling nervous about maintaining control over a group of children. The groups ranged from preschool to school-age, and targeted one specific aspect of speech or language difficulties. Most commonly, the students worked on attention and listening with preschool children, and moved on to phonology or word-finding with the older children. The preschool children attended group sessions with their parents, so the aims of these sessions were not only to improve the children's skills but to model interaction strategies to the parents so that they could implement these in the home environment. Some of the students ran group sessions several times each week and, although enjoyable, the intensity of this type of service delivery came with challenges.

> One of the challenges was the amount of children that we saw. We were seeing six children or six groups a day. There were three kids in my group sessions, then you've got three children's notes to write up. So you're kind of getting your head around one child, reflecting on the whole session, your performance, their performance, and then you're on to the next. And I did find that sometimes there was not a lot of time to reflect on each individual child. **Martina**

Many of the students also helped to run groups specifically for the bilingual children on their caseload, supported by bilingual speech and language therapy assistants (SLTAs). Vanessa enjoyed these sessions and found that, in addition to the SLTAs bringing their language skills to the sessions, they were also able to offer insights into some of the important cultural differences.

> They had so many referrals of children at the age of 3, bilingual, not talking or difficult to assess. There were six children in each group and they had a block of 12 weeks. It gave a chance to assess, and a bit of demonstration to the parents about how to play. They had a couple of bilingual [speech and language therapy] assistants. They were saying in their culture, they don't tend to do as much child-centred play. They said it was really good to show the parents good ways to get their child communicating with them. So we just did that for the first couple of hours and obviously you can imagine how much fun it was when they're 2 or 3 and tottering in. A lot of the parents couldn't speak English, so they [the SLTAs] would translate or we'd always use English first, if the child wasn't responding then they'd try and use the child's home language. Sometimes the therapist would take a back seat and do the recording of the children and let the assistants take the group. **Vanessa**

Training for parents

A small number of the students became involved in delivering Hanen training to parents (The Hanen Centre[13]). The Hanen programmes provide early language intervention lfor the parents and caregivers of young children by offering training that promotes language development and social communication skills. The Hanen Centre offers a range of programmes for certified speech and language therapists to deliver, but the students on these mainstream paediatric placements were all involved with the 'It Takes Two to Talk'® programme. This programme promotes strategies for parents to use with children under 5 who present with delayed language development. All of the students involved in this intervention were supervised by their Hanen-certified CE and only permitted to deliver a proportion of the training. Training parents was one of the most daunting aspects for the students, but those who took the opportunity had very positive experiences and felt that their confidence increased enormously.

> She [the CE] did a lot of Hanen training for parents. The first week of my actual placement we'd gone to the houses and done the initial videos of the interactions, so I got to meet half the children and the parents before, which was nice, because I knew who they were and what the kids were like. The first week I just observed the training and then the following week, she [asked if I was] happy to present some of it and I said "Not really", and she said "You'll be fine". So then after that she would ask me which section I'd like to present and I got to present a section of it. [It was] a good opportunity, because I was scared of parents and speaking to groups of people does scare me. The parents were all friendly and lovely. It was really, really good to have that experience as a student, when you're not expected to do it perfectly and have the feedback from people, like "Oh, that was really good, well done". It was quite encouraging. It was nice having an active role…to feel a bit more part of it. The parents asked me for advice sometimes and they asked questions if they were unsure, and they always fed back that they'd understood. The parents on the Hanen

---

13   The Hanen Centre, www.hanen.org.

> training were coming back each week really enthused
> and with nice feedback about the children and things that
> they'd done. **Anya**

Molly also delivered a section of the training to a group of eight parents. She was initially concerned that being young and having no children of her own may have hindered the parents' acceptance of her advice, but she found that they were very receptive and she was able to utilise some of her own experiences to gain rapport with the group.

> It was making the parents aware that you're not there
> to lecture them, it's just to help them out, and I used
> examples from my cousins or my goddaughter to make
> them see that other people find it hard as well, it's not just
> them. **Molly**

Summary

Due to the estimated high incidence of speech and language impairments among children, all of the students felt that it was vital to gain as much experience as possible of working with this population. The challenges of these placements varied according not only to the type of placement, but the confidence that individual students had in their ability to interact with children and their parents. Those who lacked experience felt that they grew in confidence over time, and many felt that they had really made a difference to the families that they worked with over the course of their placements.

> One of the little boys I saw regularly, he was such a quick
> learner and it was just amazing. You just think, "Wow, I'm
> helping you, you can suddenly say /p/ at word level when
> you couldn't before, and that's from me being able to teach
> you how it's made." And being able to help him with that
> was really good. And there was a little boy who was 5…
> he was at a two-word level, but I got him to look at a card
> and say "Cat kick the ball" and it was like, "I've done that,
> I've helped you be able to start using three words together."
> When you see something happening it's just the best thing
> ever. **Matt**

Top tips from students

- Gather resources to help young children settle into sessions, e.g., bubbles, interactive books. These are especially useful if you are working with preschool children.

- Be very familiar with norms and prepare your own list of speech and language norms that you can use as a quick reference source.

- Think about ways to maintain a child's attention during sessions. Using games as rewards works well but ensure that this does not distract the child from the main focus of the session.

- Make a list of advice for parents of preschool children about encouraging speech and language development. Print this off and be prepared to talk it through with parents.

- Put together a list of formal assessments that target each aspect of speech and language, but also think about how you would assess these areas informally.

- Consider how your approach needs to differ depending on the age of the child that you are working with.

- Provide steps up and down within session plans, but always have in mind further adaptations that could be made to tailor a session to the child.

- Work with teaching assistants and use their knowledge about the child.

- Practise phonetic transcription before your placement to improve your accuracy and speed.

- Sometimes the simplest activities are the easiest to administer and just as much fun for the child as more elaborate ideas.

Top tips from clinical educators

- Revise theoretical knowledge of early language development and norms.
- Consider the role of environmental factors on language development.
- Research the importance of using rhymes and songs to promote speech and language development.
- Be creative. Find out which toys and activities are currently popular with the age range and use these in assessment and therapy activities.
- Try to gain as much experience as possible of playing with and talking to young children prior to placement.
- Think about the feedback that you give and the purpose of this feedback, e.g., is it to praise and encourage the child, or to inform them whether or not they were on target.
- Think about your own language levels as well as the child's and ensure that your language is not too complex for them to understand.
- Wear comfortable, washable clothes because you will spend a lot of time playing on the floor!
- Compile a comprehensive list of case history questions and try to practise with your peers before you go out on placement.
- Prepare a pro-forma for classroom observations to guide you and structure your observations
- Practise transcription skills using CDs or any audio material. Make sure that you are comfortable transcribing non-English sounds as these come up frequently.
- Listen to the therapist, the child and, most importantly, the parents.

5 Dysfluency

Stammering or stuttering are interchangeable terms that describe a breakdown in the fluency of speech. Dysfluencies can manifest in a number of different ways: repetition of the same sound, syllable or whole word, blocking on sounds and sound prolongations (Enderby, 1996). Around 20% of children experience non-fluent speech, approximately 1% of whom have a stammer which persists often into the teenage years and adulthood (Enderby et al., 2009d). The evidence posits a range of factors that can contribute to the manifestation of developmental stammers. Brain imaging has revealed different levels of activity in the motor cortex of those who stammer compared to those with typical fluent speech (Watkins, Smith, Davis, & Howell, 2005), and higher dopamine levels have also been detected in dysfluent speakers (Maguire, Riley, Wu, Franklin, & Potkin, 1997). Approximately 60% of children with a stammer have a relative who stammers, suggesting a strong genetic basis in many cases (Enderby et al., 2009d). The family environment may also play a role, with factors such as high parental expectations, a busy environment and social pressure sometimes contributing to the development or perpetuation of a stammer (Enderby et al., 2009d). Stammering most commonly manifests in early childhood during the period of rapid language development. There is some evidence to suggest that a mismatch between linguistic, motor, pragmatic and articulatory abilities during this period of change may be a causative factor (Adams, 1990) and this hypothesis may also explain why such a significant number of stammers resolve during childhood as the child's language system stabilises with age and development.

Students who have a placement with clients who stammer work in a range of settings, from specialist clinics to schools, though they are usually supervised by a specialist SLT regardless of their placement location. This chapter highlights the experiences of five students who worked with clients of all ages, and illustrates that a single diagnosis does not necessarily lead to a homogenous group of clients. The students describe the different environments in which they saw their clients. They reflect on their experiences of assessing and carrying out individual and group therapy with paediatric clients, and the challenges of working with the parents of their clients. Those who also worked with older clients consider the different demands of working with teenagers and adults who stammer.

Caseload

The students worked in a variety of settings, with clients ranging from young children through to adults. Libby had a school-aged caseload and travelled to see her clients at a number of different primary schools, whereas Mysha was based in a specialist clinic and worked with clients of all ages.

> I worked with a girl who was 6 years old and then I worked with somebody who was 18 years old and then I was doing sessions with an adult, so it was a wide range. My clinical educator was a dysfluency specialist, so he saw pretty much all of the department's dysfluent clients. **Mysha**

Leila spent her placement at an integrated care centre for children, seeing clients who ranged in age from pre-school to mid-teens. She explained that although there were many different professionals based at the centre, there was very little opportunity for multidisciplinary teamwork and she worked solely with the speech and language therapists (SALTs) and assistants. Caitlin was based in a community clinic where she saw clients of all ages. Prior to her placement, Caitlin assumed that she would work solely with paediatric clients and so found the range in ages to be both the most unexpected and challenging aspect of her placement. Briony primarily saw her clients at a community clinic, but she also travelled extensively to a range of children's centres and schools. Consequently, she had to plan very carefully in terms of taking resources with her and keep accurate records of the clients and parents that she saw each day. Briony found working in the school setting particularly demanding, feeling that her clinic-based sessions presented fewer environmental challenges.

> The schools were challenging because there would be lots of other children around, and there'd be lots of screaming and it'd be quite disorientating. And then you'd have to go and find the child and you'd say to the teacher, "Which one is he?" In a clinic, they'd come to you and it was a quieter environment. In primary schools...I did one assessment with this child in a staff room and people kept coming in and out, and it was just really hard. **Briony**

Many of the students felt that lectures had helped them to develop a solid understanding of the theoretical underpinnings of dysfluency, but they were daunted about putting this into practice with their clients. For most, the nerves dissipated as they began to see their clients and apply their knowledge to real cases.

> It's all very well doing theory…but then when I saw it, it really, really made sense. So I think you need to see things for it to make sense. **Briony**

Several students were surprised to find themselves working with children who had a range of other diagnoses in addition to their stammer, but the evidence shows that the incidence of stammering is higher in some children with particular learning difficulties (Enderby et al., 2009d). In some cases, this brought about additional challenges that required the students to call on their wider clinical skills.

> It was a first session of PCI[14] [parent-child interaction] and he [the client] was 3 and had suspected ADHD [attention deficit hyperactivity disorder]. The therapist was running the session obviously with his mum there, but there was absolutely no way you could have done it with only one person in the room, because as soon as he got in through the door he was everywhere: on the chairs, climbing up to the ceiling, it was incredible. I was there as his kind of container, I think. We got through eight activities in half an hour, so that was quite an eye-opening experience, to get him to attend and interact. And obviously with quite a severe stammer it was challenging. **Libby**

The students also observed significant variation in terms of the severity of their clients' stammers. Briony helped her clinical educator to run a regular group therapy session to support primary school-aged children and felt that seeing several clients at once really illustrated the range of severity.

> Some of them had quite severe stammers, but some of them from what I could see were quite mild. I expected them all to be really bad. None of them were brilliant, but I expected them to be a lot worse really. **Briony**

---

14 Rustin, L., Botterill, W., & Kelman, E. (1996). *Assessment and Therapy for Young Dysfluent Children: Family interaction*. London: Whurr.

Three of the students had adults with dysfluency on their regular caseload. Briony found that many of the adult clients were reluctant to have their sessions observed or run by a student due to high levels of anxiety, but her work with those clients who did provide consent allowed her to gain a great deal of insight into the significant impacts that stammering can have throughout a person's life. Despite increased public knowledge and acceptance of stammering, some people who stammer continue to experience prejudice and difficulties in the workplace (Enderby & Emerson, 1995; Klein & Hood, 2004) and several of Briony's clients discussed the impacts of their stammer on important aspects of their lives.

> They spoke about emotional aspects a bit more…a lot of them weren't comfortable with having a student, which I've never experienced before…they'd not been able to find work because of their stammer. **Briony**

Interacting with clients

All of the students were initially nervous about how they should interact with a client who stammers. They were most concerned about whether to help clients who were struggling or to give them time to express themselves without intervening. Mysha explained her strategy for dealing with this situation so that both she and her client felt comfortable.

> I got them to fill out this form and it said whether they liked people finishing their sentences or not. So I always knew before I saw them. So you just have to wait…and another thing they say is to maintain eye contact…and I found that a bit difficult. When they struggled to get a word out and you were still looking at them. That was a bit awkward, but then once you got to know them, that just went and it was natural then, so it wasn't too bad. **Mysha**

Caitlin explained that it was important to show her clients that she was attentive and listening carefully. She felt that this helped her clients to feel more at ease and consequently more willing to talk about their experiences. Many people who stammer experience high levels of anxiety as they are speaking (Enderby et al., 2009d), so all of the students learned that helping clients to feel at ease was an essential skill to master whilst working with this client group.

> Give them loads of time to talk and speak. And not smiling when they're talking. I was told to not smile because they can sometimes interpret that as you laughing at them. **Caitlin**

The students who worked with teenage and adult clients recognised that their style of interaction and use of terminology needed to be adjusted so that they could engage their clients in therapy and build rapport, particularly given that some students were working with clients of a relatively similar age as themselves..

Case history and assessment

Taking a detailed case history was an important part of the students' placements and they all felt that they developed skills in this area, despite it often being challenging. Caitlin used the case history sessions to gain a deeper understanding of her clients' experiences and perspectives; however, she found that often the children felt uncomfortable talking about their stammer.

> They would look down and not pay attention. I tried techniques to [maintain] the child's attention. Saying something like, "I can't see your eyes, or are you sleeping"... stuff that was quite child-like. **Caitlin**

She also found that taking a case history from the child could be difficult if their parents were present for the session because they sometimes answered on behalf of their child. This made it more challenging to gain the child's true perspective about their stammer and the psychosocial impacts. Research has shown that parents are often very concerned about their child's dysfluent speech, whilst in many cases the child has not yet developed the same degree of insight and self-awareness (Enderby et al., 2009d). Often a case history was taken from the child and then a separate one from the parents to gain a true picture of their perceptions and concerns and to avoid parental concerns being made apparent to the child.

The case history provided information about the clients' self-perception and the impacts of their stammers on their lives. Some of the students also used more objective, quantitative measures to gain information about the type and severity of their client's stammers. Leila gained experience of assessing dysfluency based on the protocol outlined by Lena Rustin (Rustin, 1987), which provides a quantitative assessment of stammering. Initially, she observed her clinician carrying out the assessment but, as the placement progressed, she began to work more independently, asking the child to carry out tasks such as saying ten words or reciting the days of the week, whilst she counted the number of dysfluencies.

> You have a clicker in one hand and a clicker in the other. And then your left hand you click all the syllables and then your right hand you click the dysfluent syllables. So it's quite confusing but the more you do it the more you get into. **Leila**

Caitlin was one of several students who regularly used the Wright and Ayre Stuttering Self-Rating Profile (WASSP) (Wright & Ayre, 2000) to gain an insight into her clients' perception of their stammer and the emotional, cognitive and behavioural impacts of dysfluency. Although clients are able to complete the rating sheet independently, Caitlin sometimes conducted the assessment within a session and so found it useful to do some preparation in advance.

> On the WASSP assessment you have certain categories that you're going to ask the client about but you only have key words. So if you want to find out about their feelings, you need to come up with a sentence yourself. I found it difficult the first time because it had to be clear and concise…so I had to go away and write down a list of questions. **Caitlin**

Intervention

Although all of the students spent some of their time taking case histories and administering assessments, their days primarily consisted of running individual or group therapy sessions.

Intervention for children who stammer can take a number of different forms. Therapy that targets the child's environment is common, addressing the range of possible causative factors and training family members to adjust their own interaction style. Direct therapy is also common and may target the dysfluency in particular, or aim to improve speech and language skills if the case history and assessment indicate them as a possible underlying cause of the dysfluency. Most of the students carried out observations of their clinical educator during the early stages of their placement and gradually took on more responsibility for a small number of clients as their placement progressed. Others found that they were relatively restricted to learning through observation due to the use of therapy approaches that required postgraduate training. Libby found that Parent-Child Interaction therapy (PCI) (Rustin, Botterill & Kelman, 1996) and the Lidcombe programme (Onslow, Packman, & Harrison, 2003) were the most common approaches to intervention on her placement. PCI therapy addresses the environmental factors that may be contributing to the child's stammer and focuses on strategies designed to promote fluent conversation between parents and children. The Lidcombe programme takes a more behavioural approach to dysfluency and is characterised by positive reinforcement of fluent speech and strategies to avoid and cope with any dysfluent episodes that do occur (Jones et al., 2005). Libby's role in both of these therapy programmes was to interact with the child and contribute to discussions with her CE after the session rather than directly carry out the therapy. However, she did have other opportunities to administer other types of direct therapy and described her approach with a 6-year-old client whom she saw regularly.

> I was doing things like slowing speech rate control, quite a lot of video work that he'd watch back, learning to identify what type of stammer it was, it just helped him recognise it. So that kind of worked with him. **Libby**

Libby also carried out joint sessions with her clinical educator to help another 6-year-old child who presented with a stammer. Her experiences illustrate the range of ways in which children of the same age with dysfluent speech may be addressed by speech and language therapy.

> He had a much more severe stammer, totally different case management, very severe blocks, lots of anxiety issues. So [it] was more sort of counselling that the therapist was doing with him. He was very, very, self-critical, and he found it quite difficult to look for the positive things in himself. So it was interesting to see that different aspect, because they were the same age, they both had a stammer but it was completely different severity and completely different

> types of child. And he did become a lot more confident. The approach to his therapy was trying to encourage him to be positive and really, really having to emphasise the progress he made because he wasn't recognising that. **Libby**

Most of the students discovered that having a sound knowledge of the core therapy approaches helped them to design and tailor therapy programmes to individual clients. Mysha found that much of her intervention combined aspects of a variety of specific dysfluency treatment programmes rather than strictly following one prescribed approach to therapy.

> All this theory, it's good to know, because actually a lot of the techniques used with them were based on these different sorts of programmes. But none of them were followed to the bone where they could be called each one of those programmes. **Mysha**

Fluency controlling strategies such as blocking modification techniques, cancellations and easy onset speech formed the basis of most of the students' direct work with clients. Mysha worked regularly with a 7-year-old client, encouraging her to produce fluent speech using these strategies and to identify when her speech became dysfluent. She found it particularly difficult to achieve a balance between encouraging the child to persevere with therapy that she was finding challenging and moving on to new tasks in order to avoid the child becoming distressed or more aware of her stammer.

> She was trying to say something, and she goes, "Oh, I can't say it my throat hurts." I was like "That's OK, we'll try and say it again." It was hard because I didn't know whether to push her to just try and say it, or whether to leave it and move on, and you're sort of caught between the two. **Mysha**

Mysha also spent some time working on functional strategies with her clients. Prior to setting therapy goals, she found out more about whether they liked to talk to other people about their stammer or if they had particular difficulties at school, and used this information to devise functional approaches tailored to that child's experience.

If they stammered and say they had a supply teacher, they could take the card up to the supply teacher so the supply teacher knew not to necessarily put them on the spot or make them read aloud. **Mysha**

Many of the students worked with clients who achieved their therapy aims and made noticeable progress during the course of their therapy block. This was a particularly rewarding aspect of the placement because the students were able to observe the positive effects of their therapy programmes.

I think that's why I liked dysfluency, because you could sort of see immediate effects. This boy…he was sat hunched forward, and my clinical educator said, "Sit back, take a deep breath before you say something" and automatically his dysfluency decreased hugely. **Mysha**

Although all of the students regularly saw clients for individual therapy sessions, their placements were more weighted towards delivering group therapy. The groups were predominantly for primary school-aged children, usually with three to six children attending each session. Some of the groups focused on the ways that the children felt about their stammers and Caitlin found that the children really enjoyed attending these sessions because this was often the first time that they had met other children with a stammer.

They were with other people who stammered, the activities were fun, there were a lot of games. You'd talk about an issue around stammering, and then you'd have a game around it… it worked well. **Caitlin**

Other groups focused on encouraging the children to develop strategies such as restarting sentences, talking slowly and bounce starting. Several of the students used Snooky The Snail™ as a basis for their group sessions and found that this was extremely popular with most of the children.

All of the students gained some experience of either contributing to group sessions or running them independently as their placement progressed and their self-confidence and skills developed. Although this was something that made them feel nervous, they also found that running group sessions was a rewarding experience. They saw their clients' confidence in their speech increase as they began to use fluency-controlling strategies in group conversations. In turn, the increase in confidence and control of their stammer further helped to alleviate the frequency and severity of their dysfluency.

> There were a couple of kids that just wouldn't talk at first because they were so aware of it [their stammer] and had been bullied at school. But as the weeks went on they'd come up and just talk to me, and then by the end of the ten weeks they were talking to the whole group. It was really nice, you do feel like you make a difference, definitely. **Leila**

The approaches to intervention with teenage clients were often quite different, focusing on strategies, relaxation and counselling to address the more pervasive psychosocial impacts often experienced by older clients with a stammer. Leila worked with two clients regularly, with a focus on using strategies in clinic and generalising the use of these to everyday situations. Her experiences offer anecdotal support to research that suggests stammering can negatively impact education and relationships (Crichton-Smith, 2002).

> I had one that was 12 and one that was 16, that came in individually. The 12-year-old had been quite badly bullied so we did lots of confidence stuff. And the 16-year-old didn't want to do her French speaking exam for GCSE...so it was more about real practical strategies, but completely talking at their level, being completely open and honest because obviously they're aware of it and they know all about their own stammer. We went outside and spoke to strangers asking the time and stuff, and then coming back in and saying, "How does that feel"? "Did they notice your stammer?" It's kind of making them realise that it's not the end of the world. **Leila**

Mysha found that many of her older clients were more comfortable about discussing their stammer than her younger clients. Sessions with her 18-year-old client were very client-led and focused on relaxation and counselling, but she was supported and supervised by her CE who stepped in to assist if the sessions became difficult. She explained that the session plans for her teenage clients were quite different from those she prepared for her younger clients.

> When I wrote my session plan it was more generalised. So it was a chat about reading or relaxation and it was

> more just to see where it went. My clinical educator, she
> didn't specifically ask for them [session plans], I'd do them
> because I found they helped me. There was no pressure to
> set goals or anything like that. But then at the same time
> you think, "What if they don't want to say anything, how
> do I prompt more"...but actually after the first couple of
> sessions, and how open they were, [I] looked forward to
> the sessions. **Mysha**

Caitlin worked frequently work with adults clients, including a gentleman who
had developed an acquired stammer following a stroke. She also described
a client in his 20s who found that slowing his speech down and adopting a
staccato rhythm helped him to communicate more clearly.

> That was the best way for him to communicate...it was
> amazing to see, it was difficult, because you could see how
> he was struggling so much and he'd had this problem for
> so long and yet he was still trying to conquer it and find
> ways of communicating effectively. **Caitlin**

Working with parents

Almost all of the students deemed working with parents to be one of the most
challenging aspects of their placement with children who stammered. Some
found that parents blamed themselves and required reassurance about the
causative factors of stammers.

> They got really emotional, and dealing with that in an
> appropriate and empathetic way was quite challenging.
> Because obviously you know, they're older than
> me. **Leila**

Some of the students found the 'Demands and Capacities' model (Starkweather,
1987) to be a particularly useful basis for these discussions because it helped
to illustrate some of the key issues in a way that was accessible to parents. The
model provides a basis to evaluate and reduce the level of communicative
demand being placed on a child whilst simultaneously encouraging strategies
to increase fluency (Adams, 1990). Briony found that she needed to adopt a

sensitive and empathetic approach when she was working with families and needed to be reactive to a range of different attitudes and situations.

> Sometimes the parents were a challenge, they were very protective. You had to be very careful with what you said. And you had to say things like, "Oh, your family environment seems quite busy", and then they'd be a bit like, "Well, what do you mean?" That was sometimes really difficult. And then you'd play with the child…and sometimes they just didn't stammer! So that was really hard as well, feeding back to the parent, "I haven't seen your child stammer." That was a bit of a challenge. **Briony**

The students all liaised with families directly in terms of taking a case history in the initial session. The children were often then placed into groups and although these sessions were only attended by the children, most of the students interacted with their parents after the group session and provided some feedback on their child's progress.

> At the end the parents came in and the children spoke about what they'd done during that session, and they filled in a form about whether they think they know a bit more and how ready they are to leave the group…because they left when they felt ready to. **Leila**

Emotional impacts

Interestingly, the students not only talked about the emotional impacts that stammering had on their clients and their families, but also the emotions that *they* felt during their placement. Some of the students found it difficult to work with older children who were more aware of their stammers, whereas others found the social impacts on some of the younger children came as a shock.

> Sometimes they didn't want to interact with people of their own age. When we did school visits…you could see that they didn't want to and that was quite upsetting. **Briony**

The evidence suggests that people who have a stammer that persists into the teenage years and beyond often develop social anxiety and low self-esteem (Enderby et al., 2009d). Four of the students worked regularly with teenagers who stammered and felt that the challenges they faced were slightly different compared to those they experienced during their work with younger children. The students found that emotions often ran high during these sessions and often found their work with teenagers particularly demanding. Many of their teenage clients had been accessing speech and language therapy services throughout their childhood and so the intervention approaches used were quite different to those used with younger client who were new to therapy and had less insight into their stammering and the possible range of psychosocial impacts.

> I found it easier with the younger ones, but with the older ones I found it more difficult because there are a lot of emotions tied in with it. There was this one boy...he was 18, and because I didn't feel that much older than him and he was talking about all of his emotions, I felt quite uncomfortable and I think he felt really uncomfortable and he didn't want to tell me. **Briony**

Summary

The experiences of these five students illustrate the wide range of settings and clients that may be encountered on a dysfluency placement. All of the students shared the same initial concerns about interacting sensitively with their clients, working effectively with parents and putting the theory into practice. However, all of the students felt that they learned a great deal, developed a raft of transferable skills and felt as though they made a tangible difference to their client's speech.

> I know I was so lucky, I'm really, really grateful, because I actually love dysfluency now, and I really think, "Oh, I want to do this job!" **Mysha**

Top tips from students

- Make an information pack about dysfluency before you go on placement. This could contain definitions of key terminology, summaries of key assessments and descriptions of the most common therapy approaches. You can carry this with you and use it to look up information whenever you need to.

- Be aware of other possible factors that may impact or be the cause of stammering, e.g., phonology or language disorders.

- Understand the different therapy approaches, but know that you do not always need to stick to them rigidly…be flexible!

- For your paediatric clients, devise some specific terms for their stammer which will help them to understand and describe it, e.g., smooth vs bumpy.

- Ask your clients some questions to establish what does and doesn't help them: How do you feel about people finishing your sentences if you get stuck? Do you feel comfortable talking about your stammer?

- Consider encouraging your clients to use art as a way of expressing themselves if they do not feel comfortable talking about how they feel. Then ask them to describe what they have drawn. This can open up a discussion in a way which is more comfortable for your client.

Top tips from clinical educators

- Try to experience what it is like to stammer by practising stammering in public places.

- Read up on basic counselling techniques.

- Take separate case histories from the child and their parents.

- Use a 'situation ratings' questionnaire to understand which situations are the most challenging for your client. This can be used to create a hierarchy of functional goals.

- Use a true–false quiz with parents and older children as a way to discuss facts about stammering and to generate discussion.

- Take a 'solution-focused' approach. Ask questions such as, "What do you do that most helps your speech to be fluent?"

- Don't just focus on fluency. Spend time talking about good communication. Good communicators can manage their fluency more effectively!

6 Cleft palate and velopharyngeal insufficiency

The craniofacial region and oral cavity are formed between the fourth and tenth weeks of embryonic development. As the emerging components of the palate develop and fuse together at around ten weeks after conception, the oral and nasal cavities are separated. There are several stages at which this process can break down, but if the fusion is incomplete, the child is born with either a cleft palate, or a cleft lip with or without a cleft palate. These different presentations represent malformations which occur at distinct stages of prenatal craniofacial development. The available statistics indicate that these types of orofacial clefts occur in around one in every 700 live births, though it is widely acknowledged that the prevalence varies according to geographical location (Mossey & Castillia, 2003). The evidence suggests that combined cleft lip and palate is more prevalent in males, whereas cleft palate is more common among females (Mossey, Little, Munger, Dixon, & Shaw, 2009). There are genetic and environmental risk factors associated with the development of cleft lip and palate (Mossey et al., 2009). The evidence indicates that between 30% and 40% of children with cleft lip/palate also have a known syndrome (London Dysmorphology Database). Several hundred known genetic syndromes include cleft lip and palate as a feature, the most common of which are Pierre Robin Syndrome and Van der Woude Syndrome (Gallagher & Berg, 2012; Howard & Lohmander, 2011; Mossey et al., 2009). Environmental risk factors include exposure to tobacco, alcohol, viral infections and particular types of medication during the early stages of pregnancy (Gallagher & Berg, 2012; Mossey et al., 2009).

Oral and nasal speech sounds can only be produced accurately if there is adequate airflow and air pressure, and if the oral and nasal cavities can be closed off by the velum. Coordinated and accurate muscle movements are required for the velum and pharyngeal walls to open and close the velopharyngeal isthmus, which enables intelligible speech production. Velopharyngeal insufficiency

(VPI) results from inadequate closure of the velopharyngeal isthmus, leading to two key speech symptoms. A hypernasal tone occurs particularly on vowels, and nasal air emission occurs during consonant production (Enderby et al., 2009a).

Surgical intervention varies widely, even within the UK. The World Health Organisation has issued a set of guidelines for the delivery of craniofacial surgery and care (WHO Human Genetics Programme, 2002), although there remains little consensus in practice, both in terms of the types of surgical procedures that are carried out and the optimal timing of these procedures (Howard & Lohmander, 2011; Peterson-Falzone, Hardin-Jones, & Karnell, 2010). The aims of surgery are to repair the cleft so that the oral and nasal cavities are separated by the hard palate, whilst avoiding atypical maxillary growth and enhancing speech sound development (Leow & Lo, 2008). Surgery on the soft palate enables efficient velopharyngeal closure and these changes to the anatomical structure of the region have a positive impact on speech development, feeding and hearing. Surgery may consist of a single operation, during which both the soft and hard palate are repaired, usually when the child is between six to eighteen months old (Enderby et al., 2009c; Howard & Lohmander, 2011). Two-stage procedures are also common. Typical practice consists of a soft palate repair between three and nine months, followed later by the hard palate closure anywhere between twelve months and early adulthood (Howard & Lohmander, 2011). This variation reflects the 'trade-off' between allowing optimal craniofacial bone growth and providing the client with the anatomical adjustments necessary for intelligible speech.

Four students had a placement with clients who had a cleft lip/palate or VPI. Three of those students worked in the acute hospital setting, and one spent his placement working with children in the community following their discharge from hospital. These placements reflect the journey that most children who are born with a cleft or VPI take during the early stages of their lives: from pre-operative assessment and surgical intervention, to therapy and regular reassessment of speech until early adulthood. This chapter describes the experiences of students in the acute setting, in terms of their caseload and the multidisciplinary approach to treatment. The students primarily carried out speech and feeding assessments whilst providing advice and reassurance to both the clients and their parents. The chapter then highlights the experiences of one student who worked alongside a specialist link therapist in the community, where the emphasis moved away from assessment to focus much more on direct intervention.

The acute setting

Caseload

Three of the students spent their placements in the acute setting, working with children who had a cleft palate, cleft lip and palate, or velopharyngeal insufficiency (VPI). The hospital setting meant that the students gained experience of working with clients who were at a range of stages in their journey, some of whom were inpatients having surgical procedures, others who attended outpatient clinics for assessment and intervention post-surgery. Cleft provision in the UK is provided by a team of highly specialist professionals, including specialist speech and language therapists who offer assessment and support to children and their families during the journey from diagnosis to post-operative reviews. The UK hosts a number of regional Specialist Cleft Centres, where staff also liaise with community clinicians (Enderby et al., 2009c). Three of the students were based within these specialist hubs.

Debbie worked in a cleft assessment clinic, primarily working with children who had undergone the second of their two-stage surgical intervention to close the hard palate cleft. Her clients ranged in age between 5 and 12 years old. Some had undergone surgery very recently, whereas others were attending the clinic for longer-term follow-up assessments. She also spent some time observing other specialist clinics to experience the full range of service provision for these clients.

> There was the cleft feeding clinic…and I got to sit on the craniofacial clinics. Then there was the cleft clinics, which was talking them through the surgery that [was] coming up to or that they'd just had. **Debbie**

Leah joined the cleft lip and palate team at a specialist paediatric hospital, where she also worked with clients with VPI and other craniofacial abnormalities. Many of her clients had speech impairments and dysphagia as a consequence of their clefts or VPI. Charlotte also worked as part of a specialist cleft team at a hospital, where they received around 80 new referrals each year from the particular region of the UK. She described the types and timing of the surgical interventions carried out in this particular service.

> The palate revision surgery [was carried out at] about 18
> months. There are no set guidelines in terms of what is the
> best optimal time. Within the unit, they had certain ideal
> times in terms of when the best results were [achieved]
> in terms of the repair. And then [the client] would have
> an alveolar bone graft at about 9 [years old], because the
> jaw has to be sufficiently mature and the dentition has
> to be right, which is why there is a lot of orthodontic
> involvement. And then any further revision, for example
> rhinoplasty, doesn't occur until about 17, because of adult
> growth. **Charlotte**

An alveolar bone graft is a common procedure for children born with a cleft
palate, and is usually performed when the child is between 8 and 10 years old.
The alveolar ridge, between the upper teeth and hard palate, often develops
with a cleft that requires repair to allow development of the teeth. All of the
students found that a basic understanding of the different types of common
surgical procedures was essential to help them meet the needs of their clients
and their families. Charlotte found that clients tended to have their initial
surgery at around 18 months old, but then returned to the cleft assessment
clinic at regular intervals for a range of assessments and reviews with different
members of the MDT.

> Generally it would be 18 months, 3 years, 5 years, 8 years, 11
> years and 15 years old. It's a process for life…you're allowed
> to re-refer yourself at any stage. But generally if everything
> had been done in terms of primary and secondary and any
> revision surgery, they [would] be discharged at 15 [years
> old] on the basis that [they] could come back at any time,
> should a fistula appear, or [if they] wanted some further
> revision [surgery]. **Charlotte**

Working in a multidisciplinary team

All of the students discussed the highly specialist nature of their placements,
and the factors that made this particular placement quite different to those
that they had experienced previously during their degree. They agreed that
one of the initial challenges was the amount of unfamiliar medical terminology

that they were required to understand and use, but all of the students quickly developed this skill by revisiting lecture notes and textbooks and by working regularly within the multidisciplinary team (MDT). The MDT consisted of a range of highly specialist professionals, many of whom SLTs would not typically work with outside of the cleft setting.

> There was a team of four speech and language therapists, of Band 7 and higher. They worked very much as a multidisciplinary team with the consultant plastic surgeons, audiology, orthodontics and psychology. In the morning [we would] tend to have a joint consultation clinic…so you would see around six to eight children in conjunction with the consultant plastic surgeon. **Charlotte**

The students relished the opportunity to work closely with and learn from professionals with such expertise in their field. Charlotte expected there to be more of an hierarchy within the MDT, but found that everybody contributed to discussions and all perspectives were taken into consideration when planning intervention for clients. Leah particularly enjoyed the intensity of being part of an MDT and seeing her clients regularly.

> I really enjoyed being in hospital with children. The team work around the child, you get that when everybody's in the same place, everybody's working together. You're involved from the beginning to the end. It's more intense, we were going up [to see clients on the ward] every day. So it's more involvement with the children, whereas in the community it's once every now and again and you don't feel like you're making as big an impact as you could. **Leah**

She attended an MDT meeting every morning to discuss the clients on the ward. Each professional outlined their planned input pre- and post-surgery so that all team members understood the care plan. She explained that the child's parents then attended the later part of the meeting and each team member explained the planned course of action. The hospital environment was, however, not without its difficulties and some of the students found that working as part of an MDT was one of their biggest personal challenges on this placement.

> The biggest challenge for me was the multidisciplinary working…you are liaising with some very highly specialised, very well educated, qualified consultants, audiologists [and] radiologists who really know their stuff. I think given the multidisciplinary nature, [you need to] be professional all the time…suss it out and know how to pitch yourself. It's very much reading the situation, reading the people and adapting. **Charlotte**

Many of the students felt that their clinical educators acknowledged the specialised nature of the placement and offered them high levels of support and encouragement to reduce any potential anxiety, particularly during the early stages of their placements. Despite initially feeling daunted by the prospect of working with such specialist clinicians, Leah soon grew used to the environment and was given the opportunity to observe some of the surgical procedures first-hand.

> By the end of [the placement], the surgeon offered me a day in surgery. There was one child who had a full cleft lip and palate, and [it was] very wide…basically the whole roof of the mouth had gone. It was just the initial repair, the first surgery. And then there was another one which was even wider and it all seemed to go wrong…and I was panicking thinking, "He's not going to be able to fix this", but he was fine and carried on and tried a different thing and fixed it in the end. It was hard having to concentrate for five hours…but it was good! **Leah**

Working with parents

The students found that due to the young age of most of their clients, they liaised regularly with parents or guardians, both when the children were inpatients and when they came into the hospital for outpatient appointments. One of the main challenges was to explain the likely impacts of cleft and surgical intervention on speech and feeding development in a way which parents could understand, whilst at the same time providing reassurance and not adding unnecessarily to the level of concern from parents about their child. Leah found that most parents had lots of questions, and that she was not always qualified to answer them. She addressed these situations by ensuring that she knew who to put the parents in touch with so that their concerns would be addressed.

> I found that parents were very, very worried, wanting something to be done straight away. The speech therapists seemed to be the first person they came across because that was the initial assessment…it was being able to have the knowledge to answer the questions without saying that that's definitely going to be the case, because we weren't qualified really to say for sure…it was quite hard to get that across to parents. **Leah**

Charlotte worked in a regional specialist cleft centre and many of the clients and their families had travelled from across the region to attend appointments. Based on her previous experience on placements, she questioned the impacts of clients needing to travel long distances to attend appointments, but soon found that this was not an issue.

> The parents, almost without exception, tended to be very motivated, very few DNAs [did not attend], compared to community clinic. About ten years ago when they decided to specialise the unit, one of the concerns was that people had to travel so far [and] that would be a big turn off. In fact, that was never, ever given as a reason. People just didn't mind [travelling] because they were getting specialist help. So I actually found them incredibly motivated. **Charlotte**

The students liaised most frequently with parents prior to surgical intervention and in the period immediately after the cleft repair. Leah understood that parents often found it difficult to make decisions on behalf of their child about whether to proceed with surgery, but was still often surprised about the reactions of some parents and found it challenging to simply provide the information and guidance without influencing their decisions based on her own opinions.

> It was surprising, you would get some parents who would come in with a child who [had] all sorts of strange articulatory behaviours where you were thinking, "Something needs to be done"…some parents [said], "Well, I can understand him and he's doing alright and I'm not sure I want to put

him through the surgery"…we would be thinking that [surgery was] definitely the right route to go down. Then you would get other parents that had a child that maybe had a little bit of nasal emission or just a bit of a grunt in the nose and they wanted loads of surgery straight away. So there were very different reactions from parents. Some of them surprised you the way they didn't want anything to be done and others the opposite way. Nobody can be forced to send their child to surgery, but it was just a case of showing them the pros and cons…telling them about what the future would hold if the surgery was withheld from them [the child], or what would happen if they did have the surgery. Sometimes it was hard not to say, "I think you should do it". **Leah**

The students also supported parents after their children had gone through surgery, providing advice about feeding and speech sound development in the weeks following the procedure.

At least once or twice a week we'd go up on the wards to see the children who had just had surgery to see how they were…they'd had the surgery in the afternoon and then we'd go up the next day. [We would] also discuss with the parents any concerns they had, just to make sure they were clear on what they needed to do post-surgery. **Charlotte**

The students had a range of emotional reactions to their placements. Whereas some did not feel as though they were particularly affected by the situations, Leah found her placement difficult in this respect. Many of her clients presented with cleft palate or VPI as one element of a genetic condition that had additional impacts on the child and their family. This may go some way towards explaining why she often found her particular placement so demanding.

I think I'd prepared myself for it to be quite emotionally charged and to be upset, looking at some of the children and listening to the parents. If you put yourself in that situation you could let yourself get really upset. But the trick was not to show any of that concern to the people in the situation. I would come home and get all upset about it, but nobody else seemed to…it was the norm in that situation. Everyone just spoke about it so matter of fact. I think once I got used to that, it became easier. **Leah**

Assessment

Despite being based in different locations, the students consistently reported that their placements were heavily weighted towards assessment of their clients as opposed to carrying out therapy. The most commonly-used assessment was the Great Ormond Street Speech Assessment (GOS.PASS) (Sell, Harding, & Grunwell, 1994), adopted by all students to assess speech sounds pre- and post-surgery. The GOS.PASS is one of the most widely-used assessments in the UK of the types of features associated with speech production in cleft and VPI. It is a comprehensive assessment, which particularly examines the phonemes likely to be affected and allows information to be collected about resonance, nasal emissions and the craniofacial anatomy. A more detailed phonological inventory can also be assimilated using sentence repetition from the GOS. PASS and the students usually carried out the whole assessment with their clients during the initial assessment session prior to surgery.

> If there was any sort of cleft palate or VPI, then you would definitely be involved and tend to do a speech sound examination using the GOS.PASS. So you would listen to all the speech sounds and also for resonance as well, dysphonia, hypernasality or hyponasality. And then you'd discuss it with the consultant plastic surgeon. The number of times you do things by very nature you become happier doing it. So I felt very accomplished at doing a GOS.PASS. I felt a lot more comfortable in my phonetic transcriptions… specifically in terms of nasal emission, nasal turbulence, have they got any oral pressure consonants…it was a lot of phonology work. **Charlotte**

The same assessment was carried out after the post-operative swelling and pain had reduced, in order to document any immediate changes in the child's speech. The GOS.PASS would then be administered at subsequent review appointments to measure the impact of speech work carried out at home with parents or via a community therapist. During the initial stages of placement, both Debbie and her CE transcribed and scored the GOS.PASS so that she could practise her transcription skills and compare her scoresheets to her clinical educator's results. This gave Debbie the confidence to develop her skills and she soon felt able to administer the assessment and oral examination independently. Phonetic transcription was one of the key challenges cited by the students, particularly because the children usually presented with unusual phonological processes and poor intelligibility.

> You really couldn't understand sometimes what the children were saying at all. And it was frustrating for them, as well as that you were trying to assess them…tuning your ear in to all the different sounds. I knew that it was going to be a lot of phonetic transcription, so I had tried to brush up on that, but it is completely different listening to phonetic CDs when [somebody is] purposefully making sounds which you're tuned in to which are said between 'ah', and them coming out in spontaneous speech. Even the same sounds can sound slightly different depending on which child was saying them. Me and the clinical educator would sometimes get slightly different transcriptions, and I [thought], "Is that because I'm completely off the target?" [Usually] we were very close and it was individual judgement. It was difficult, because so much was riding on the assessments that are perceptual and if people are making slightly different judgements…it wouldn't make that much difference to what would happen, though. They were normally very similar and meant the same thing, so those small differences didn't matter but that really bothered me at first. I was panicking that I was doing it wrong all the time. It took me a long time to start tuning in as well, I only felt more confident right at the end of the placement and I was constantly feeling like I couldn't do it. Whereas at the end my clinical educator said we were surprised at how quickly you picked it up. So I think they do recognise how difficult a task that's going to be. **Leah**

In addition to administering the GOS.PASS with most clients, the CLEAR phonology screening assessment (Keeling & Keeling, 2006) was also used by several students to take a phonological inventory. Leah explained that she would usually carry out the most appropriate assessment followed by a case history from the child's parents prior to surgery. All of this information was then fed back to the other team members at the MDT meetings.

Charlotte carried out regular ward visits to work with children and their parents during the initial stages post-operatively. This was an unexpected element of the placement for Charlotte, who had assumed that she would only see clients in outpatient clinics at the hospital.

> We were checking the notes to find out exactly what repair had taken place, because sometimes the surgeon wouldn't know exactly what he was going to do until he got in there. So [we] needed to check exactly what surgery had happened. And then it was a matter of trying to assess the child's speech the day after. Sometimes they [the children] were so grumpy with us that they wouldn't cooperate… and they were very sore and groggy. They were around 18 months [old]. We just really wanted to hear if there was any hypernasality. Ideally, they would be hyponasal, because they'd be really blocked up and swollen. So I would say primarily it was really to reassure the parents and to do follow-up for them. We'd have to explain to the parents that actually we'd gone from one extreme to the other and as the swelling went down we were hoping for somewhere in the middle. **Charlotte**

In the weeks after surgery and discharge from hospital, the client and family would attend the outpatient clinic to discuss the range of therapy options available. These ranged from home programmes for parents to administer, referral to a community SLT for local provision, or a short intensive block of therapy at the regional referral centre if this was convenient for the family.

Intervention

The students carried out only a small amount of direct intervention during their placements. This was in part due to the specialist nature of the work carried out primarily by highly specialist therapists, and in part due to the way some of the services were run. In some instances, the SLTs in the hospital were responsible for the assessment and family support immediately pre- and post-surgery, and clients were then referred on to local services for intervention. One of the consequences of this was that some students found it more difficult to build rapport with their clients and their families and cited this as one of the downsides of this type of placement.

> There was little continuing contact with the same client. The vast majority of it was reviews. There was only one client that I saw for three sessions of therapy, and that was interesting because that was an on-going client for one particular SLT. She worked with a little girl to try and get placement of the tongue prior to her cleft being repaired. And then we saw her in the ward afterwards and she [the child] wasn't happy with us at all. And then we saw her two weeks later. [They] have a sort of two week hiatus…they don't go to school and have a soft diet. Then we saw her in clinic after the two weeks for another couple of sessions, and she was really starting to use the sounds. But other than that one occasion, I don't think I saw the kids or the adults more than once. That was one of the disadvantages of the placement, because there wasn't that opportunity to see the process through. I followed the process through but with individual children at different stages. **Charlotte**

Debbie was able to carry out some direct intervention during her placement. She primarily worked on articulation and feeding, two of the key difficulties for children with a cleft palate or VPI. In terms of speech prior to surgery, children with cleft palate commonly experience articulatory difficulties specifically with sounds that require high oral pressure (Chapman, Hardin-Jones, Schulte, & Halter, 2001), such as plosives, due to the inadequate separation of the oral and nasal cavities. They also present with difficulties producing palatal and alveolar sounds due to their atypical oral anatomy (Trost-Cardamone, 1990). Although feeding difficulties vary depending upon the type and severity of the cleft, common issues include poor oral suction and pressure, nasal regurgitation and coughing or choking (Morris & Klein, 2000). Children who have difficulty feeding often require bottles with teats that have specific adaptations to the shape, opening or pliability and allow the child to gain adequate nutrition (Kummer, 2008).

> We ran a baby babble group before surgery...so it was
> sort of a pre-emptive strike to get the babies making the
> shapes so eventually when they did have that closure, the
> /b/ would come out or the /p/. The feeding clinics were
> to do with the bottles...just basically going through the
> different bottles. With the cleft, they can't get the suction,
> so it was just going through that with the parents if there
> were any difficulties. **Debbie**

The community setting

UK cleft services are organised so that there are clear links for liaison and collaboration between the Specialist Cleft Centres and community speech and language therapists (Enderby et al., 2009c). The RCSLT states that the regional specialist services function as hubs of expertise and provide advice and support for local therapists (Enderby et al., 2009c). Charlotte spent each morning carrying out joint consultation clinics with inpatients, and then either ran one-to-one articulation therapy sessions in an outpatient clinic based at the hospital, or accompanied her CE on school visits. During the school visits they would meet the community link therapists who would be taking on the children as part of their community caseload following discharge from hospital. The therapists and Charlotte would then work together to run joint assessment and intervention clinics. Although Leah did not work directly with the community therapists during her placement, she observed her CE liaise regularly over the phone to provide advice to clinicians who were not specialists in the field. She also regularly wrote case notes and reports about her clients which were sent on to the clients' community SLTs. During her time on placement, Leah found that she assessed many children who had been referred from the community due to a suspected cleft or VPI, and noticed that often the referrals were not appropriate.

> The amount of referrals which were wrong...it was nothing
> to do with the cleft lip and palate or VPI. It was learned
> behaviours, which seemed a bit like it could be a cleft lip or
> a cleft palate type characteristic. If there was a bit of nasal
> emission or a nasal grunt, they were being referred straight
> away for specialist assessment. And you'd assess them and
> you'd do the GOS.PASS, check for airflow...and it would not

> be that [cleft or VPI] at all. Then they had to write back and say that it was not a cleft type characteristic, they thought it was an articulation and learned thing... [they would] write back to the therapist with what sort of therapy techniques they want them to do and have quite a lot of involvement with the community therapist. And then if there was still no progress and they were concerned, they'd refer back again. They did see a lot of people, but it was surprising how many shouldn't really have been referred. **Leah**

Luke had a very different experience on his cleft placement, working with a clinician in the community setting. His CE had a mainstream paediatric caseload, but was also a cleft specialist and acted as a link between the acute and community settings. Luke's experiences highlight the range of speech and language therapy provision for children with cleft lip/palate and VPI, and illustrate the different roles that clinicians fulfil in this specialist field.

> We did a fair bit of travelling so we didn't see many patients in the day. She had quite a big caseload...on her own she maybe had 40 that were just cleft, and then above that she had more that were mainstream phonology. It was mainly kids in schools, we took them out of their lesson and did therapy with them. All of the kids that I saw were post-surgery, all a couple of years on and still having [regular check-ups]. They were kind of between maybe 3 and 7 [years old] and in mainstream schools. **Luke**

Unlike the students based in acute settings, the focus of Luke's placement was direct therapy with his clients. Despite this difference, he faced many similar challenges to his peers, and agreed that phonetic transcriptions were a particularly difficult aspect of his placement.

> There was lots of transcription. Even just really basic stuff like places of articulation...but when you're put on the spot...and also some phonetic transcription really got me, all the extra IPA[15] stuff, all the other bits that aren't just phonemic things were really useful to know, because lots

---

15   International Phonetic Alphabet, a system of phonetic notation.

> of the noises they were making weren't typical, and we had to get all those down as well. **Luke**

The intervention that Luke carried out primarily focused on developing clients' articulation and phonology. Children with cleft lip/palate or VPI usually present with hypernasal resonance, nasal air escape and articulatory problems (Enderby et al., 2009c). Although most of the therapy approaches used by Luke were comparable to those used for any children with articulation disorders, there were particular sounds which were common among his client group and the methods employed in therapy were adjusted to suit the fact that his clients usually had a high level of insight into their own articulatory difficulties.

> Lots of /s/, that tended to be the big one that they couldn't get their heads round, and nasal [and] bilabial sounds. The kids were very, very aware [of their speech difficulties] and we did lots of work in mirrors. Because they were so aware of it, they knew a lot about it and what they needed to put where [in terms of place of articulation]. They all seemed to grasp the concept really, really well. [One client] was 4 and she knew exactly what she was doing looking in the mirror and looking at me and tucking her lip under. **Luke**

Almost without exception, Luke worked with his clients at school. Home visits were rare and, unlike the students based in hospital settings, he had little contact with the children's parents. More frequently, he liaised with teaching assistants and provided them with exercises to carry out with the children throughout the week.

Summary

Placements in this area of speech and language therapy are highly specialist. Although some students felt that they were not able to gain as much direct practical experience as on placements with other client groups, they were extremely positive about their experiences and were able to reflect on the range of transferable skills that they developed.

> I wasn't really sure what to expect, but it was really interesting and I really enjoyed it! And as a specialism I found the whole thing very interesting. **Luke**

Top tips from students

- Read as much as you can about the different types of cleft lip and palate and VPI. Make sure you understand the biological basis of the formation of cleft and VPI and how these will look on observation.

- Read in detail about how speech is likely to be affected, often known as 'cleft type characteristics'.

- Know about the syndromes that are most commonly associated with cleft.

- Really understand the GOS.PASS (Sell, Harding, & Grunwell, 1994) assessment. Learn how to administer and record by practising before placement.

- Make sure your phonetic transcription skills are up to scratch! Practise the more unusual sounds on the extended IPA chart, but remember it is never as easy to identify these sounds in a real life setting. Do not get upset if at first you struggle to identify speech errors or make accurate transcriptions.

- Recognise that the placement can sometimes be emotionally draining.

- Use your instincts to judge when it is an appropriate time to talk to parents.

- Prepare yourself to be working within an MDT and discussing cases with other professionals on a regular basis.

Top tips from clinical educators

- Revise and retain age norms for speech, language and general development, particularly for the ages of 18 months, 3 years and 5 years because these are the most common ages for assessment or reassessment of speech.

- Do some background reading on cleft palate and understand some general terminology. Your clinical educator will not have a big expectation of detailed knowledge.

- Learn about hypernasality and nasal emission.

- Revise the relevant anatomy, particularly the hard and soft palate.

- Turn up on time, dress professionally and show enthusiasm!

- Be aware of the common assessments of phonology and articulation for children.

- Familiarise yourself with the GOS.PASS and read the journal article that outlines the development of this assessment (Sell et al., 1994). Watch the associated training DVD if it is available.

- Keep a copy of the extended IPA to hand and brush up on diacritics.

- Don't forget that you will have skills that are transferable from previous placements, e.g., case note writing, case history taking, writing reports.

7 Children with complex needs

'Complex needs' can manifest in many different, highly individualised forms. Children may present with difficulties from birth, or they may develop during the early years subsequent to injury or illness. Complex needs are often associated with the diagnosis of a life-limiting or lifelong medical condition that affects communication or swallowing, including autistic spectrum disorder (ASD), Down's syndrome, Duchenne muscular dystrophy, cerebral palsy and global developmental delay. These varied conditions can cause difficulties with motor speech, voice, language, communication and swallowing. In addition, children commonly present with co-morbid impairments such as sensory deficits, learning difficulties, challenging behaviours and motor impairments. Many children with complex communication needs operate at a preverbal level (Goldbart & Caton, 2010), using modes of communication such as eye gaze, pointing, gesture, facial expression and sometimes vocalisations.

Children with learning difficulties often require special education provision, which comes in many forms. Some children receive additional support in mainstream education from the special educational needs (SEN) team, others attend language units attached to mainstream schools and some attend specialist schools. Special educational needs coordinators (SENCOs) work with the child, their parents or guardians and teaching staff to provide individual education plans (IEPs), which outline the targets, strategies and provision for a child (Department for Education and Skills, 2001).

In this chapter, five students recount their hugely varied experiences on placement with children who had a wide range of complex needs. They discuss the environments in which they saw their clients and the impacts of these settings on their sessions. The routes for referral, types of assessments and most common diagnoses formed a major part of the students' reflections on their experiences. The students talk about the most common intervention approaches used with their clients and their feelings about working with the parents or carers of the children.

Setting

Whilst some students were based in one location for the duration of their placement, others combined home visits with regular sessions in specialist schools. This creates a complex picture, demonstrating the variety of experiences and challenges faced by students, often within a single placement.

Alex spent her placement in a range of primary schools that catered specifically for children with different levels of learning disability. She spent one day each week at a school for children with mild-to-moderate learning disabilities, and another full day based in a school for children with profound and multiple learning disabilities (PMLD). Alex spent the rest of her week working with children who were receiving specialist services for their complex needs in a mainstream school setting and she occasionally visited clients at home. The most common diagnoses that Alex's clients presented with were autistic spectrum disorders, Down's syndrome and global developmental delay. She helped to manage a large caseload of children, and on a typical day would carry out both individual therapy sessions and some group therapy. Alex typically worked with five to ten clients each day and also spent time liaising with teaching assistants at the schools. Some of the major challenges of the busy school environment were finding rooms in which to carry out her sessions and maintaining her appointments whilst being adaptable in her approach:

> It really made me realise how flexible you need to be, because obviously children have different lessons, sometimes they have lessons that they shouldn't really miss, but then you're at school only from 1 until 3 or 1 until 2, because you have another appointment. I think it really made me realise how flexible you need to be, and you always need to think…if I can't see this child, can I see somebody else? You know, just to use the time, not to travel for nothing. **Alex**

She found that the links between speech and language therapy services and the schools were generally very good and that regular communication between the different professionals led to a very effective service for the children. Alex worked closely with teaching assistants at each of the schools and developed a much greater understanding of their role and the way in which speech and language therapists could liaise to support the children within the classroom setting:

> I really came to appreciate the role of teaching assistant. Before, I thought they just supported children, helped them during their class. I wasn't aware that they actually carried out the therapy to the extent they did. It was really important to listen to their experiences, because they are with these children all the time. I observed some really great cooperation by the SLTs and the TAs. **Alex**

Jade spent her placement at a school that catered specifically for children from the age of 4 years old with PMLD and sensory impairments. Many of her clients had a diagnosis of ASD and co-morbid visual and hearing impairments. She usually ran one small group session and three one-to-one sessions with clients each day, although this varied depending on the medical stability and challenging behaviours of her clients and she needed to take a flexible approach to planning her days at the school. Niamh carried out regular school visits throughout her placement, but she also spent a significant amount of her time making home visits to work with both children and their parents. The majority of her clients presented with ASD, Asperger's Syndrome, or behaviour profiles that indicated one of these possible diagnoses. Operating as part of a multidisciplinary diagnostic team is a common role for speech and language therapists who work with young children presenting with characteristics of ASD (RCSLT, 2006) and this was a key part of Niamh's role on her placement.

> They [the clients] were generally aged between about 2 and 16. We did some home visits, which were assessments to see whether the children would be appropriate to have a diagnosis [of ASD]. We did school visits, which again were to see if we could find any features of ASD to contribute towards a diagnosis. And others were checking on [therapy] programmes [and] to see how the environment was for the child. So we visited some mainstream schools...some were units within mainstream schools, and a lot of the units had mainly children with ASD or global delay. And we also visited some specialist ASD schools, the pupils there were aged between 3 and about 16 and again that was more assessing, setting programmes for teachers. They all had a diagnosis in that school. It was very varied, some assessments but some intervention as well. It was a bit of everything really. **Niamh**

Niamh felt that she was able to gain a deeper understanding of her clients during school visits because she was able to observe and assess the children engaging in a range of different activities. She carried out classroom and break time observations, and was also able to engage with their parents at the end of the school day to gain further insight and provide feedback. Home visits proved to be a more challenging setting for Niamh.

> On a home visit, you've not really got that opportunity…it's only one environment. And I think on a home visit, a lot of the information that we were getting…we were having to rely on what the mum was saying or the dad was saying, we could only make minimal observations. Whereas in a school, we could actually back up what our opinion was with things we'd observed in different settings, which made it a lot easier to actually put towards a diagnosis. **Niamh**

Nadia was based in a community clinic for her placement with pre-school children with complex needs. Although some of her clients already had a diagnosis of ASD, Nadia primarily worked alongside other SLTs as part of the multidisciplinary diagnostic team:

> Quite a few of the children hadn't been diagnosed [with ASD], and so they came to us at the clinic or we saw them at home or at nursery. Then we would attend meetings with the GP and with people from the EarlyBird group. And the parents would attend as well. Then we would discuss [a] diagnosis. **Nadia**

The EarlyBird programme was created by the National Autistic Society to support the parents of pre-school children who have a diagnosis of autism, helping them to understand and manage the key symptoms (www.autism.org. uk/earlybird). Although some children were diagnosed at a pre-school stage, Nadia learned that often the MDT preferred to wait until the child was slightly older before making a diagnosis of ASD. Like Niamh, Nadia found that home visits often raised the most challenges, particularly if the child's siblings were present during the sessions. She found that taking extra materials for the sibling to play with independently helped the sessions to run more smoothly.

> A lot of them had a younger sibling in the room who would just crawl all over everywhere. That was quite a challenge.

> Getting used to keeping them [the sibling] occupied but
> not letting them interfere with the session. They just
> want to do whatever the child that you're working with is
> doing. **Nadia**

Lily had a somewhat different experience on her placement with children,
working in a specialist children's hospital as part of a highly specialist team
of SLTs. She initially found the demands of placement were overwhelming,
but she observed and worked with a very large number of clients and soon
developed an understanding of their wide range of needs.

> It was a bit daunting at first…there was so much to learn
> about the different conditions and about the process that
> children go through when they're investigating…when they
> suspect that it's a genetic disorder…where they get sent to.
> In the first couple of weeks I thought my head was going
> to explode, but then by the end of it I was quite surprised
> by the depth of my knowledge. I loved the setting. Because
> you've got the inpatients and outpatients, so you've got that
> variety. You're also seeing the progress…from them coming
> in, [through] to discharge…I [worked with clients who]
> had craniofacial abnormalities, paediatric dysphagia, I did
> cardiac feeding clinics…I learned all about heart conditions
> and the effect that they can have on feeding. I just found
> the whole thing just completely fascinating…It was just a
> huge learning experience for me. **Lily**

In addition to working closely with the speech and language therapists, Lily
interacted regularly with other professionals both on the wards and within
MDT meetings. She felt that this was an important aspect of her placement,
both in terms of providing high-quality client care and in aiding her own
professional development.

> I think it was good seeing the multidisciplinary teamwork…
> it was such a big team. That was really useful and it gave me
> the confidence to be able to speak to different professionals.
> Obviously you first go in and you've got all these surgeons
> and you're a bit intimidated. By the end of it I'd got to know
> them quite well, it gave me the confidence to ask more
> questions. **Lily**

Referral, assessment and diagnosis

Niamh and Nadia primarily worked as part of the team who were assessing children for the triad of characteristic features of ASD: impaired social interaction; communication impairments; and stereotyped behaviours (World Health Organisation, 1994). Nadia found that most of her pre-school clients had been referred into the service either by nursery staff or by parents, usually due to concerns about a lack of social interaction with their peers. Niamh observed a similar pattern of referrals, but also discovered that health visitors had often identified atypical developmental patterns and referred their clients for further investigations. She found that the traits of ASD were often not recognised until the children started school.

> The youngest was about 2, there were a lot of features [of ASD], it wasn't so difficult to spot the diagnosis, it was very plain to see. I think the oldest was about 5 or 6 and he was more towards the Asperger's end [of the spectrum]. So, whereas his parents had just thought he was slightly eccentric, the school had picked it up, because they'd previously had children with a similar diagnosis. **Niamh**

With the exception of Lily, the students found their placements were heavily weighted towards assessment as opposed to carrying out direct therapy, an aspect that was a surprise to many. Some clients required an informal approach to assessment, whereas others were assessed extensively using a range of different formal assessments. Alex found it challenging to carry out informal observations during the early stages of her placement, though her confidence increased with experience.

> It was a bit of a challenge for me at times, with children with PMLD, to adjust to the way you look at things with them, because you need to go back to such a basic level... it was informal observation, partially based on P-levels[16]. I think you really need to be flexible with how you think about things. During my first day I was thinking, "What am I looking for?" Sometimes these are things that are difficult to find in books because you need the practical experience of how to look for an eye gaze, how to interpret

16   Qualifications and Curriculum Authority. (2009). *The P Scales.*

things, are they actually intentional [communication] or
not? **Alex**

Niamh also found observational assessment a challenging aspect of her
placement, but soon realised that learning as much as she could about the
features of ASD helped her to differentiate these from the typical behaviours
displayed by age-equivalent children. All of the students who worked with clients
on the autistic spectrum were surprised by the huge range in severity of the
characteristics that they observed among clients with the same diagnosis.

> Going in and having presumptions about autism was
> something I struggled with…the fact that not all children
> with autism are the same. I expected them not to let me play
> at all with them, not to speak to me, I think the severity of
> it was what I wasn't expecting…the range, the spectrum.
> I wasn't expecting that. But it was just through lack of
> experience I think, and obviously you can read a book,
> but seeing it is completely different. **Nadia**

Niamh also worked with children from across the autistic spectrum. She
found that the outcomes of a parent questionnaire or assessment could be
very different depending on the particular constellation and severity of
symptoms exhibited by each child, but still indicate a diagnosis of ASD on
different points of the spectrum. She also discovered that often the accounts
from nursery about a child's language and cognitive development could be
quite different to parental reports, highlighting the importance of accurate
assessment in addition to taking a comprehensive case history from as many
different sources as possible.

> The reports from parents and reports from nursery were
> quite different. There was one parent that we spoke to and
> he didn't think that his child could say ten words and when
> we did a language sample he was actually really shocked,
> and he was apologising to his son because he'd not believed
> that he could say that much. **Niamh**

The students administered a wide range of formal assessments, some to assess
the core domains of speech, language and communication and others to aid in
the diagnosis of a child with traits of ASD. The Test for Reception of Grammar
(TROG) (Bishop, 2003) was used by several students to assess their clients'

understanding of different grammatical constructs, the Renfrew Action Picture Test (RAPT) (Renfrew, 2003) was used to assess expressive language and the Pre-School Clinical Examination of Language Fundamentals (Pre-school CELF) (Semmel et al., 2006a) was used to assess both the receptive and expressive language abilities of particularly young clients. The South Tyneside Assessment of Phonology (STAP) (Armstrong & Ainley, 2012) was the most frequently-used phonological screen; however, several students also used the Diagnostic Evaluation of Articulation and Phonology (DEAP) (Dodd et al., 2006) to provide a more thorough examination of articulation and phonology. Niamh and Nadia both used the Autism Diagnostic Observation Schedule (ADOS) (Lord et al., 2012) and the Symbolic Play Test (Lowe & Costello, 1988) as part of their assessment battery for children with a suspected diagnosis of ASD.

The ADOS (Lord et al., 2012) is a semi-structured assessment battery which examines communication, social skills and imaginative play in order to quantify the client's performance in terms of the triad impairments of ASD. Nadia used the Symbolic Play Test (Lowe & Costello, 1988) to assess the development of her young clients' imaginative play and symbolic awareness, both of which are key indicators for early language development and are often areas of difficulty for children with a diagnosis of ASD (Enderby et al., 2009b). Many of the students practised these formal assessments with their peers prior to carrying them out with clients, and felt that their skills in terms of administering the assessments had improved as a result. Despite this, Alex found that sessions did not always run as smoothly as planned and that a flexible approach was vital.

> I had one girl who I was doing the STAP with, and she was sitting next to her mum and she was just so overwhelmed… it might have been because I was a new person. She just wanted to be with her mum all the time, and then she was putting her hand into her mouth all the time and she would just say "No, no". So it definitely helped to look at it [the assessment], but at the same time you need to be prepared that you might have to think on the spot. **Alex**

Intervention

All of the students engaged with a range of different types of service delivery. In addition to individual, direct therapy sessions with regular clients, most of the students also ran group sessions and designed programmes to be carried out by teaching assistants in the classroom setting. Several of the students used Picture Exchange Communication System (PECS) (Frost & Bondy, 1994) or the TEACCH approach (Treatment and Education of Autistic and Related Communication Handicapped Children) (Schopler & Reichler, 1964) as a basis for their therapy. PECS is a picture-symbol system which originally aimed to aid children with ASD to engage in transactional exchanges of communication (Bondy & Frost, 1994). It is now used more widely with a range of clients who have complex needs, but the premise of encouraging the child to exchange a picture-symbol for the object that they want remains the same. The TEACCH programme was developed at the University of North Carolina by Dr Eric Schopler and colleagues in the 1970s. It is an educational strategy designed to promote the independence of children with ASD, using highly structured visual support systems. Although primarily an educational strategy, elements such as visual timetables and colour-coded systems are often adopted by speech and language therapists to promote communication, and many specialist schools in the UK follow the TEACCH approach. Niamh spent her placement in a school that used TEACCH principles in the classroom, and found that it was important to understand the system in order to engage with both her clients and the school staff.

> Make sure you know PECs, the TEACCH system, communication books, visual timetables. A lot of the time, you might go to a session and it's not been documented that the child uses PECs or that the child uses TEACCH and you'll be expected to integrate that straight away. So make sure you have a basic knowledge of it, so that if you are thrown into that situation you can just think, "Right, OK, let's slot that in." **Niamh**

Intensive Interaction (Nind & Hewett, 1988, 1994) was the most common therapy technique used with clients who had PMLD on Alex's placement. This approach is widely used in the UK to encourage client-led interaction (Goldbart & Caton, 2010), aiming for frequent and meaningful exchanges to promote joint attention and social communication (Nind & Hewett, 1994). The exchanges between the client and therapist are often nonverbal signals such eye contact, physical proximity and mirroring, though echolalia can also be used with verbal clients.

> I had my first Intensive Interaction with one child and it was going nowhere. I don't know if it was partially me, but [the client] was not reactive, she was doing her own thing and I was trying to copy and look at her and be playful. And then I had another Intensive Interaction with somebody else and actually I felt a connection and it was pretty amazing…you realise you just sometimes need to put a little bit more effort. **Alex**

Jade also found that Intensive Interaction was a rewarding way to engage with clients who presented with profound disabilities and sensory impairments.

> If you got a child to engage in eye contact with you who is operating at pre-intentional level and is suddenly holding your hand or reaching out or giving you an object, asking for more…I got a 'more' request with one student and I came out skipping. That's enormous, you know. They're tiny, tiny, tiny steps but they're so important. They're so crucial and that's the difference you can make. **Jade**

The students found that their placements generated a great deal of reading and their sessions required careful planning. The highly specialist nature of Lily's placement in the children's hospital meant that she spent a particularly significant amount of time reading about unfamiliar medical conditions and the associated speech, language and communication difficulties. Lily only worked with one client regularly, a 4-year-old boy with Duchenne muscular dystrophy. Her sessions focused on expressive language and Lily found that, although challenging in many respects, her experience was highly rewarding.

> I loved my sessions with him, but it was quite sad…obviously I had to learn all about his history and and he'd been in hospital pretty much all of his life. I think she [CE] had been working with him for quite a while and he'd never said a two-word phrase. I got 'more fish' out of him and it was the best thing. He was quite hard to keep motivated and he was quite hyperactive so that was a challenge. **Lily**

The students all described specific clients whom they had worked with regularly throughout their placements. Jade's experiences illustrate the multitude of complex needs with which her clients presented.

> I worked with an 11-year-old who had the most complex needs. You know when you just sit in the room and go, "OK, I haven't got a clue what to do here." But I got there in the end. He was operating at the pre-intentional level, he had cerebral palsy, attention deficits, oral fixation. Really bad seizures, so you'd work with him and it'd be going really well and he'd have a seizure and then you were back to day one. Massive attention difficulties. So I was working on eye contact, joint attention and sensory stimulation and Intensive Interaction with him. **Jade**

The complex and specific needs of clients often included sensory impairments, which needed to be taken into consideration when planning therapy sessions. There is a great deal of evidence to suggest that hypersensitivity to stimuli such as light, sounds and textures is a pervasive feature of ASD for many children (Enderby et al., 2009b). Alex liaised regularly with OT and physiotherapy to find out more about her clients physical and sensory requirements, and Niamh agreed that this kind of information was vital in helping her to carry out effective sessions.

> Use little pieces of information to your advantage. I had a child who was really interested in fire extinguishers. If you know a piece of information like that, you put that into your sessions, because that's really going to help you in delivering the session. Any type of motivation that you know they will work towards, use it. That should be one of the first things you're asking a teacher or a parent... "What will motivate them?" And, as well, if they've got any issues that aren't necessarily speech, language or communication...like sensory issues. Some of the children didn't like the sound of paper being folded or scrumpled. That can completely ruin your session. You need to be very aware of all behaviours, not only the ones that are related to speech and language. **Niamh**

Many of the clients that Lily worked with had dysphagia amongst their range of complex needs. Although she was not able to play a particularly active role in the management of dysphagia, she learned a great deal from shadowing her CE and was able to carry out supervised client observations.

> The feeding side of it was a big surprise to me. I didn't realise how involved we were until I went on placement…a lot of it was feeding. Although we get taught about dysphagia, I'd never seen it on a placement. I just thought it was amazing, what they were able to do for the children. I think it was me being naïve, presuming I'd be working on their speech, but more than 50% of the placement was dysphagia. **Lily**

Most of the students spent a significant amount of time outside of their placement devising activities and games through which they could meet the session aims whilst engaging the child with therapy. Feedback from her clinical educator coupled with observations of other SLT sessions led Nadia to adjust her approach, adopting simpler approaches to maintain client engagement and to meet the sessions aims.

> With all the children, doing games with bubbles was just something really easy that you could start with and you could finish with as a reward. Doing games like, "I want you to pop the bubble on your nose"…seeing if they know the body parts. That was just so simple to use…I was over-thinking tasks. My clinical educator was just wonderful with doing such simple things and not over-complicating it and the kids still loved it. **Nadia**

The students all found that planning therapy sessions was a challenging aspect of working with children who have complex needs due to the level of flexibility required. They spent a great deal of time designing activities which could be adapted on-line during sessions to suit the child's needs.

> [I had a] lot of step up, step down activities in session plans. In assessment sessions, rather than take in one assessment, I'd take three or four…and there were cases where I did have to go through three or four assessments to find the one that they would cope with. In previous mainstream clinics where I'd maybe plan four activities in a session, I'd have to plan eight to ten to handpick which ones to use. So just a lot more thought had to go into planning really. **Niamh**

Jade found that many of her clients varied significantly from day-to-day in terms of their ability to attend to therapy sessions. She would sometimes work with a child for 30 minutes one day, but a session the following day with the same child may only have lasted for five minutes because of challenging behaviours or lack of engagement.

> I think it's really challenging, really challenging. You have to be prepared for behaviours that you wouldn't expect in a mainstream clinic…the kids are not necessarily going to do what you want them to do. So it's you that needs to be flexible, that's the main thing. Be very, very flexible. **Jade**

Alex and Nadia both developed a high level of insight into their own interaction skills and the impact that their style of interaction could have on clients. Alex ensured that she gave her clients plenty of time to process information and respond; however, her CE explained that children with attention difficulties often respond more positively to sessions carried out at a faster pace so that they can remain focused on the activities. One of the aspects that she found most difficult was establishing a rapport with some of her clients.

> I found it really emotional and quite difficult…mainly because you don't get a lot of feedback [from the clients]. It might sound silly, but if you smile to a child and the child smiles back, or you say something the child speaks back to you…obviously that makes it easier. But I think it's just sometimes a bit more difficult because you don't always feel this connection. **Alex**

Nadia also had some concerns about her interaction style, and initially found it difficult to pitch her sessions because of the tension between enabling a client-led session and ensuring that she remained in control of her sessions.

> At first I struggled with getting a balance between following their lead and doing what I had planned for the session, because I was too concerned with upsetting the child. But as it went on, I felt like I gained what I wanted from the session, but with following the child a bit as well, I got a nice balance from it. **Nadia**

Working with parents

The students all had some contact with the parents of children they worked with on their placements. Nadia and Niamh both worked directly with the parents of young children who were undergoing assessment as part of the differential diagnosis procedure. Nadia gained a great deal of experience in taking case histories from the parents of pre-school children with a suspected diagnosis of ASD.

> Quite a few of them [the sessions] were initial interviews. I spoke to the parents, while my clinical educator played with them [the client] on the floor. Then the next time we'd swap over, so she'd do the interview with the parent and I'd play with the child and observe the child. Quite a few of the parents were concerned. But then you'd get others who were like, "Why are we here?" They were always very helpful but one thing that I did struggle with was the feedback to a parent or a teacher after the session. I never knew which bits were important, and I found it really hard to make it concise and tell them what they needed to know. **Nadia**

Niamh found that revising her phonetic transcription skills and being confident about developmental norms helped her to provide more accurate and appropriate feedback to both parents and her clinical educator about her clients. She found it particularly challenging to deal with the emotions of parents who were struggling to come to terms with their child's likely diagnosis and the potential implications for their child.

> There were a few occasions where we did school visits and would see the children, then we'd also see the parents. There was a standard questionnaire that we'd go through…a checklist almost. You would have to feedback at the end of the session to the parents and a lot of the time, if there were features [of ASD] there, then we would have to say we'd be happy to put together something to go towards a formal diagnosis. It was really difficult. A lot of them got very emotional…even during questionnaires when you're not giving them any information, they're just giving it to you…that was really draining actually, how upset some of them got. **Niamh**

Niamh and Lily both felt that they were able to discuss difficult sessions with their clinical educators and felt very well supported in terms of the emotional demands of their placements. Lily regularly interacted with parents of children who were acutely unwell and often on the intensive care unit (ICU). She found that her role as a student was particularly difficult in these circumstances and she often took a step back so that her CE could lead the discussions.

> You have to use your own judgement as to whether it's the right time to talk to them [parents]. I remember there was one we went to see and the parent was deaf and the speech therapist knew a bit of sign language but not loads. And I made my own decision to sit back because it was going to be hard enough, and the baby was quite poorly on ICU. I didn't think it was really appropriate for me to go over to try and explain that I was a student. You could also tell from what was going on with the child. If they were really poorly, I'd just sit and stay quiet. But if it was just a check-up and they were doing quite well then that was a lot easier. **Lily**

Summary

Despite feeling daunted by their placements, the students all learned a great deal from their clients and their clinical educators. The complexity of each child's needs meant that it was particularly important for them to adopt a flexible, individualistic approach; skills which are vital for working successfully with any client group.

> I had never really had a lot of contact with people with special needs...I was a bit nervous..."What will I do, will I have to behave differently?" I think my placement made me realise that you just need to be still yourself and they are just people like everybody else and they have totally different characters. **Alex**

Top tips from students

- Try to be yourself and focus on the client, not on your own fears. This will help you to establish a better relationship with the client.

- Accept that first impressions of a client can be quite unnerving and daunting. It can take a long time to get to know your client and find out what works best for them.

- Be imaginative and flexible and, most of all, let them lead the work that you do with them.

- Remember that this client group comes with complex issues that are not just related to communication.

- It is vital to communicate with those who work with the client on a daily basis as well as other professionals in the MDT. This will help you immensely in terms of understanding your client.

- Make sure that you realise that ASD is a spectrum! Not every child will present in the same way and your assessments and interventions need to reflect this.

- Prepare yourself emotionally. It can be emotionally challenging to work with some children, and also parents who may be upset.

Top tips from clinical educators

- Be flexible. Although session plans are important, it is unlikely that clients will follow them perfectly. Having the confidence to alter plans within the session is critical when working with this client group. In addition to step up and down activities, plan some 'side step' activities…a different activity to achieve the same aim.

- Have a detailed knowledge about preverbal language development. This helps with assessment, observation and therapy planning.

- Have some knowledge of P Scales (Qualifications and Curriculum Authority, 2009). Many of the children are functioning at the pre-National Curriculum level and some knowledge of these levels is important because speech and language targets are embedded within each client's individual programme.

- Do not be afraid to ask for support or supervision for complex cases.

- Be as honest as you can with parents. Listen to them and think about the types of support that they could access.

- Consider children's sensory needs and preferences and how this may affect their presentation in sessions.

- Wear comfortable, washable clothes because you are likely to spend a lot of time playing with children on the floor. Keep jewellery simple because some children are attracted to bright shiny objects!

- Some of the children have complex physical and medical needs or may be unwell. We can all find this hard at times, so be honest with your clinical educator about how you feel.

8 Young offenders with speech, language and communication difficulties

Speech, language and communication difficulties experienced by young people involved in criminal activity have only recently been explored in any depth. There is strong evidence to suggest that communication difficulties are highly prevalent among this population of young people (Bryan, 2004), but the evidence is complex and multifaceted. Much of the literature examines speech, language and communication needs (SLCN) in the context of behavioural issues, mental health and learning disabilities, with evidence only recently emerging that specifically pertains to SLCN. There is a small but increasing number of specialist speech and language therapists within the field (RCSLT, 2009) and, consequently, more students are spending their placements within this sector.

Three students were interviewed about their placements with young offenders. They discussed the unique settings in which they worked with a varied caseload of clients. The types of assessment and intervention that they carried out often differed very little from the work that a student would do with any young clients with SLCN, however the context and environment clearly influenced the experiences that all of the students had on these placements.

Setting

There are over 100 youth offending teams (YOTs) in the UK that support and supervise people under 18 years old who have either been convicted of a crime or are deemed to be at risk of carrying out criminal activity. They were set up following the Crime and Disorder Act (HMSO, 1998) and although they have a wide remit, their overarching aims are to reduce the risk of young people in the community committing offences and to provide support and rehabilitation to young people following their release from a secure centre. Two of the students worked full-time with a local YOT, and the third split her time between the YOT and one of the Her Majesty's Young Offender Institutions (HMYOI) for offenders aged between 15 to 18 years old.

YOTs are multidisciplinary, though only some have a speech and language therapist and most are not full-time members of the team (Nacro, 2011). Callum and Julia worked in central YOT offices alongside legal case workers, social workers, nurses, police officers, support workers and a speech and language therapist. The students were primarily based in the YOT offices where their clients attended for appointments, though they did see some clients at home or at school on occasions. The open-plan YOT offices were conducive to MDT working, and although there were no regular MDT meetings in Julia's setting, she found that the professions all shared information about the young people they were working with in the community.

> Everywhere you went somebody was asking you about this case, or that case. So it was more informal and you talked to who you needed to, when you needed to. But then a couple of times a week, people would get together… maybe the health team around the child, or if there was a complex case, they got together and discussed a complex case. **Julia**

All of the clients that Keira worked with in the community setting had an electronic tagging order and a curfew, meaning that they had to stay at a known address between particular times and adhere to a set of conditions. Each client had an individualised supervision plan, which aimed to promote rehabilitation and reduce the chances of reoffending.

> They [the clients] would have to come in or sometimes [we would] do home visits. It depended on their tagging order or if they had a curfew, but they also had schedules and they'd have to do a certain number of hours a week. So they would either have to meet with their YOT worker or they would have to go and do an anger management course, or some kind of building course or educational course, or they'd have to go and see the nurse. So they had hours that they had to make up of contact [with particular support services] . And for some of them they'd see a speech and language therapist, so they might come and see us for an

> hour and then we would decide whether it was worthwhile building speech and language therapy hours into their programme. **Keira**

Clients who breached the conditions of their tagging order or supervision plan could be taken into custody, or recalled to a secure youth custody centre. Consequently, clients who did not attend speech and language therapy appointments were reported to the relevant authorities by Keira's clinical educator. Keira found that attendance was largely very good, but that she needed to be particularly aware of any friendships forming between clients attending the centre and report these to her CE.

> You had to monitor people's relationships...so because there were a load of boys coming to the same place, similar appointments, they would start hanging around with each other. Two young boys that were 12 and 10 had started kicking about together and they [the staff] had to start changing their appointments so they wouldn't come into contact **Keira**

Unlike Callum and Julia, Keira had a split placement because her CE had a split post between the YOT and a young offenders institution (YOI). She describes the protocol that she needed to follow each morning.

> Usually, I'd have to get there for about 8.30 and then have to go through security checks in the morning. But they weren't as bad as I thought they were going to be...basically it's just making sure that you don't have anything on you like stamps, excess amounts of money, mobile phones, keys... you don't take any of that in. And I would get picked up by one of the staff, either my clinical educator or another person in the department, because I didn't have keys so somebody would have to come and get me. **Keira**

Although this environment was completely unfamiliar, Keira explained that she adjusted to the protocols very quickly and felt well supported, not only by her CE, but by all of the staff within the secure centre.

> If you had sessions, you'd go through to their unit and pick them up. I would always have to be accompanied by

somebody. You're never left alone with them [the clients] either. There were two specific rooms that were used for therapy, but you'd always have prison staff outside the door, and the door was always open…every single room is filmed. There were certain things…like you should never have necklaces round your neck, your ID badge had to be snapable. Thinking about how many pens you went into a room with, making sure you're coming out with that [the same number]…not turning your back on somebody. But you get really used to it, it becomes second nature really quickly, and then you kind of don't feel like you're in a prison. I thought I would have a lot more attitude [from the clients]. I thought [there would] be a lot more behavioural issues and I didn't experience any of that. Because there were so many people around it was safer than you usually ever feel. If anything, probably I think the prison guards probably scared me more but I wasn't ever really scared of any of the boys. There were so many things [safety procedures] in place it just gets shut down straight away. **Keira**

Keira worked with a very wide range of professionals within the YOI. Multidisciplinary team meetings during the initial few weeks of her placement helped her to gain a better understanding of the different roles within the staff team and to learn more about the young offenders that she was working with. During the later stages of her placement, Keira was encouraged to play a more active role in these meetings and to contribute her own knowledge about the clients that she had been working with. She found that most staff had some understanding and training in communication difficulties and this was often a discussion topic during these weekly meetings.

Usually [one morning each week], I would attend a whole prison meeting. So you would go and talk about cases that were either people who were high risk of either being bullied or offending in prison, or people who were mental health risks. So they'd talk about possibly moving them around the prison, and that would involve everyone…the head of the prison, the head of wing, mental health staff, speech and language therapy staff, psychologists, everyone. You'd hear a lot of confidential information there, you would hear

everything about possible crimes that the kids had done and
you would also hear about possible crimes that were taking
place in the prison. It was quite explicit information and
would seem quite shocking because people would discuss
it…it was quite normal for them. So anybody who'd been
involved in the care or had contact with one of the prisoners
would say their opinions on what their assessments were
or how they'd seemed…so everything gets logged. In the
MDT meetings [we would] discuss new prisoners. So every
new prisoner who came in, everyone talked about how they
seemed to be settling in, if they knew anybody else, and
that's when people brought up [issues like] "He doesn't seem
to understand when I give him instructions." **Keira**

Confidentiality was also a serious issue facing all of the students on their
placements with young offenders. Although this is the case with all placements,
it became particularly complex because the students often worked with a large
number of different professionals, all of whom had different levels of access
to information about the client. Keira was guided carefully in this respect by
her CE, who came to be her main source of support because she was unable
to discuss her placement with others.

There were people in there [the YOI] who were in the news,
so you knew exactly who was who, and because they were
underage they couldn't be named in the news. Confidentiality
was such a strange thing, because lots of people would ask
you how your day would be, and you definitely didn't tell
people about it. I didn't talk to my housemates about it.
And my parents would always ask "How was it?" and I'd
be like "Yes it's fine" but that was it. **Keira**

Caseload

The students worked predominantly with male clients aged between 14 and
19 years old. There were female clients on the YOT caseload, but they formed
a smaller proportion. Young offenders' institutions in the UK are single-sex,
and Keira was based in a centre that catered solely for young males. Within
the YOI, the offenders were separated according to age, so that the younger

boys were not able to mix with the older offenders. The speech and language therapists were based on a unit with other healthcare staff such as nurses and mental health workers. Keira explained that there was a caseload of approximately 50 clients within the YOI, but felt that this number would have been much larger had there been more service provision allocated to the YOI. In the community YOT, she discovered that almost every young person under the care of the team was accessing speech and language therapy input. The nature of working between the community and custodial services in the same geographical area meant that Keira often saw the same clients in both settings as they were detained and released.

> We actually only dealt with people who were on tagging orders. So they'd either been in [a YOI] and come out and had a tagging order, or they hadn't been in and they were on tag, and basically if they offended while on tag, they went into prison. The first boy I ever worked with, we saw him and he'd been in and out of [a YOI] three times. He went to meet the lady he'd offended against and he was so positive when we met him. My clinical educator gave me the background on him and said, "He's so different this time". We did stuff about how he felt about his speech, and he was like "Yes, I really want to sort things out this time". By the time I'd left he was back in (a YOI), and I saw him when I was on my way to somewhere else in the prison...I saw him when he was on his duties and it was so strange, he couldn't look me in the eye. **Keira**

Research suggests that speech, language and communication difficulties are far more prevalent among young offenders when compared with the general population (Talbot, 2010). Approximately 60% of young people within the youth justice system have significant communication problems (Bryan, Freer, & Furlong, 2007), though some studies have suggested that more than 70% of those known to youth offending teams present with below average communication abilities (Crew & Ellis, 2008; Hamilton, 1999). Links between speech, language and communication needs and behavioural problems have been well-documented (Humber & Snow, 2001), though they are often not picked up or easily recognised within this population due to the interaction of several complex factors (Nacro, 2011). There are also well-established links between poor communication skills and mental health problems

(Linares-Omara, 2005) and research has suggested that one-third of young people with SLCN develop mental health problems, sometimes leading to involvement in criminal activity (Clegg, Hollis, & Rutter, 1999). Figures suggest that only a minority of prisons and YOI screen new offenders as a matter of course (Talbot & Jacobsen, 2009), so SCLN are rarely recognised and subsequently not addressed. Keira's experiences echoed the findings that suggest there is often a complex interaction of factors that commonly impacts on communication amongst this population.

> There was a lot of getting the boys to talk about what they had issues with, it was really mental health based. So there was a lot of "Do you get angry or frustrated when you're doing this?" and that kind of thing. A lot of the boys had undiagnosed ASD, ADHD, really low level language skills, a lot of boys were illiterate as well and that was a common thing within their family. A lot of familial-based things as well…they'd talk about problems that their parents had, or brothers and sisters would be having. **Keira**

The students all talked extensively about approaching their initial sessions with clients without any preconceptions and without judgement. They felt that this was extremely important from a moral standpoint and also felt that it helped to build trust, which led to more beneficial interactions.

> I think you need to leave your prejudices at the door… everybody was treated as an individual and not as this person who's committed this crime. People didn't come in escorted by police or anything like that. **Julia**

The students did acknowledge that leaving behind their preconceptions was not always easy to achieve, particularly during the early days of their placements when the environment was still unfamiliar and they were in the early stages of getting to know the young people they were working with during sessions.

> I suppose you can't help but have preconceptions, but just have a really open mind…I think that's the thing, don't assume anything. At the end of the day, they're still people who need help, no matter what else they've got going on. **Keira**

The level of information that the students had about their clients' backgrounds and the offences that they had committed varied greatly. Sometimes they would know more detail about clients from MDT meetings or if the client disclosed information to them; however, all of the students were advised to move conversation onto other topics if their clients discussed the reasons why they were within the justice system.

The students were all highly aware of the links between SCLN and behavioural issues and consequently expected that learning to deal with poor engagement and attention would be a significant aspect of working with their clients. However, they were all was surprised by this aspect of their placements and found that most clients were cooperative with therapy.

> They were all really well behaved, which is not what I expected. They were so open, they saw the speech and language therapist as somebody who was on their side, because they were usually the person who got things done. You know, if there was something going on that was bothering them…even things like having eczema and they were scratching…they would often tell the speech therapist because that would be the person that they felt they could just chat to. I never had anybody say anything [negative] to me, they were all very kind of, like, "Good morning, Miss" and if I walked passed they'd all say "Hello". A lot of the time they were actually happy to go to therapy because they got out of classes. Or if you did manage to get them out of their cell, depending on what the wing staff said, they'd like the fact that they get time out. So a lot of them actually were, like, "Are you coming to get me today?" **Keira**

Julia was also surprised that the levels of engagement during sessions were so high and attributed this to the approach that she took with clients.

[Sometimes] they couldn't be bothered...[but] you'd get that with adolescents in any setting wouldn't you? I did an assessment by myself in a special school and the SENCO was next door in her room and she said, "You did really well to not get a single swear word out of him". She said normally he'd be kicking and screaming as well. But she said, "I think that's about the way you approached him, you were understanding and he trusted you." We were there to help them and I think a lot of them knew that. There was no kind of abuse or anything like that. You need to relate to that person...really get down to the young person's level and be approachable basically...appear as someone they can talk to. There needs to be that genuine desire there too, I don't think that's something you can fake really. **Julia**

The students felt that both lectures and background reading had provided them with a sound knowledge base about SLCN in the youth offending population. As the students gained a greater understanding of their clients, many reflected on the possible effects of their earlier childhood experiences and the links with SCLN, behavioural difficulties and criminal activity.

When you dig deeper, you understand why these kids are the way they are. You understand why they won't trust an adult...maybe because they have not had that role model. If you dig deep, you do find out about the psychological aspects. **Callum**

The students' families and friends tended to be less well-informed about the client group and some expressed concern about the students undertaking their placement. Due to confidentiality, the students were unable to discuss much of their placement with friends or family, but their experiences suggest that they felt extremely safe throughout placement.

My partner didn't want me to do it, he didn't like the idea of me working in that environment. I think he had the stereotypical view of you're a girl in an environment with a load of boys. Honestly, none of them said anything to me, and if they did say anything of a sexual nature or any kind of innuendo, I'd been informed that I would have to

> tell people so they [would] get reprimanded. Actually, they were really nice to me. And I'd have my lunch in there as well, so if some of the boys were on cooking courses, [they] cooked the lunch for the staff or would work the tills…it was run with [a local] college. So you'd see all of them and they'd be like, "Hello, Miss, do you want the same as last week?" Socially, I think they all had so many strong points actually. **Keira**

Although every student acknowledged that their placement had some degree of emotional impact on them, they all felt that they were highly supported by their clinical educators and often by many of the other staff on the MDT. Julia felt that she managed her placement well because she had some voluntary experience within the sector, whereas Callum found it more difficult to 'switch off' at the end of a day. Keira found that she often reflected on the provision for young people with SLCN within the youth justice sector and was able to discuss her feelings with her clinical educator.

> It seemed a strange system that they probably had better care and better access to care in there [the YOI], than they would in the community. And a lot of them had similar patterns of behaviour. Nearly a third of them were fathers and then a lot of them had been in the care system for a long period of time, and had either been kicked out of school or been in behavioural schools. It just seemed bizarre that things could go that far and they still hadn't had a proper diagnosis. It did feel like a lot of those boys could have been helped a lot earlier and never been in that situation at all. And I think that's what frustrated me, the lack of provisions for people in the first place. And it just seemed so crazy that you're getting to it when it's spiralled out of control. I don't begrudge the people I was working with. There wasn't any of them that I thought…"I don't want to have anything to do with you", I didn't really ever feel like that. **Keira**

The caseload that Keira describes is relatively representative of the young people within the criminal justice system. Research indicates that speech, language and communication impairments that persist into adolescence can have a range of significant and long-lasting impacts on young people. Many leave school early following a period of non-engagement (Bryan et al., 2007; Humber & Snow, 2001) and the impacts of communication difficulties often manifest as disruptive behaviour. SLCN can cause frustration and boredom if the young person is unable to understand language, which is often incorrectly perceived as lack of cooperation leading to further issues. Julia described her session with one client shortly after he had been interviewed by the police, which clearly illustrates the potential for misconception.

> We did always ask "what happened?", and they'd say things like, "I couldn't remember what I was going to say" or "It gets muddled up". There was a boy, who in his police interviews had said, "No comment, no comment, no comment", and then when asked why by the speech therapist, he said because things muddle up when he says it, he says one version and then another and then another... in court, people start questioning why it's not the same. But that's to do with his sequencing. **Julia**

In recent years, there has been a surge of interest and knowledge about the specific links between SLCN and young people in the criminal justice system. A growing number of studies have shown that a high proportion of young offenders have particular difficulties with producing coherent, logical and sequential narratives (Humber & Snow, 2001; Snow & Powell, 2005), something that they are required to do throughout police interviews and court cases. Comprehension of complex and abstract vocabulary often proves challenging (Crawford & Bull, 2006); again, an aspect of language that is critical during legal proceedings. The links between SLCN and criminal behaviour became very clear to the students throughout their placement as they gained a deeper understanding of this complex area.

> I just love the fact there's so much that can be done. The fact that so many offenders have speech, language and communication needs and they're falling through the net at school and being labelled as behavioural problems. And then it's like finally they come to us and somebody realises the fact that their language needs can affect so much... problem solving and consequential thinking...it makes sense why they do go out and commit crime. Consequential

thinking…just that term in itself…no wonder they're offending if they can't weigh up the consequences. So I think you just view them as a person, not as an offender… how has their language got them into trouble and how can we meet their needs. It heightened my desire to work with adolescents just because it all made sense, about how language had such huge impacts. There was one boy who'd been arrested. He'd got an intensive supervision order, so he had to go into the youth offending offices 25 hours a week as opposed to custody. He was about 17, he'd left school, he was going into college. But he'd been removed from his parents' care and spent the last year of his life in foster care. He'd been told to go to the job centre, fill in all these forms, get all his benefits and things like that in place. And then he'd been involved with [a crime] so he came through to us, we assessed him and he had the vocabulary level of a 4-year-old and language levels of a 7-year-old. He had no awareness of how to fill in a form to claim any benefits. [This is] somebody whose language has really got in the way of their everyday life. **Julia**

Often the young people gained hugely from the insight that the students were able to give them into their communication difficulties. There is evidence to suggest that communication impairments in adolescence can have a significant impact on self-esteem and confidence levels (Fergusson, Horwood, & Ridder, 2005). This can lead to social withdrawal which in turn can trigger mental health problems (Linares-Omara, 2005). The students found that many of their clients were relieved to find out more about their SLCN and work with somebody who could help them to improve their communication and interaction skills.

I think they were really happy to realise that they weren't thick. That was the common thing, they were all like, "I was just crap at school, I'm thick". And it was actually, "Not that we're making excuses for you, but you find this really difficult and that's not your fault". And I think that's the first time any of them had been told it's not their fault and they all really wanted to know what that meant and what they could do about it. There were so many other things going on in their lives, they were kind of like, "I've got court coming up this week" or they had girlfriends who were going to have children and they'd have family issues… so there'd be a lot of things that'd change their mood quite drastically. But with some of them you did feel like you were changing their self-esteem which I think was the biggest thing. **Keira**

Assessment

The students used a combination of formal and informal tests to assess their clients' language skills. Although Callum carried out very little direct work with clients, those he did work with were part of an early intervention strategy that targeted young children deemed to be at risk. He worked regularly with a 5-year-old boy in a school setting, and used the British Picture Vocabulary Scales (BPVS) (Dunn et al., 2009), sections of the CELF (Semmel et al., 2006b) and the Test of Abstract Language Comprehension (TALC) (Elks & McLachlan, 2007) to gain information about the child's language development. The CELF is designed to assess the receptive and expressive language skills across a wide range of ages, and Keira also regularly used this comprehensive language assessment with her clients.

The main assessment we used was the CELF…it depended on why people had referred them, but if it was a language issue, then it'd always be the CELF, and that [language difficulties] was the main thing that we saw. We'd use that [the CELF] for reviewing as well, if there was going to be somebody coming up for parole or coming out. It was long, but with the boys it was really good because we'd be like, "We just need to get through this, let's just do this one". But if they had challenging behaviours [or] if they were just like, "I really can't be bothered", then you're like "Alright, what's on your mind, what's going on?" So it's very much like a counselling thing…if they were willing to speak to you, then you just dealt with it. **Keira**

Julia worked with her CE to train other members of the YOT to identify children known to the team with possible SLCN. She found that this was a very effective model of service delivery, which meant that she and her clinical educator could spend their time assessing those children and overseeing intervention in a school setting.

> About 99% of referrals [from other members of the YOT] were valid, so we'd assess them usually with the CELF[17] or the BPVS[18] and some informal assessment that would either be carried out at the youth offending offices or in school. And then we would put programmes into school, so it was quite school based. **Julia**

Julia and Callum did find that some clients were either not able to engage with formal language assessments, or not willing. The complexity of these clients in terms of the interaction between SLCN and behavioural difficulties made it very difficult to ascertain the reasons behind any instances of non-compliance. However, the students found that informal assessment often gave them the necessary information without the difficulties that formal testing could bring about.

> You can't really do formal assessments. They [the clients] don't really respond particularly well…not all of them, but a lot of them don't respond to formal assessments, so we were doing informal…problem solving, consequential thinking, cause and effect…that type of thing. **Julia**

There is evidence to suggest that many young people become adept at masking their communication problems (Nacro, 2011) in order to take the focus away from their specific difficulties. This is something that Keira experienced with one particular client who was very resistant to engaging with formal language assessment. As she encouraged him through the test, she found that his reaction suggested he had some insight into his own difficulties and knew that he would find the assessment challenging. This highlights the value of formal assessment in some cases and suggests that forming good rapport and taking a sensitive approach with clients is vitally important in order to gain a true measure of a client's speech, language and communication needs.

---

17 Semmel, E., Wiig, E.H., & Secord, W. (2006b). *Clinical Evaluation of Language Fundamentals-4 (CELF4)*. London: Pearson Assessment.

18 Dunn, L.M., Dunn, D.M., Sewell, J., Styles, B., Bryzyska, B., Shamson, Y., et al. (2009). *British Picture Vocabulary Scales-3 (BPVS-3)*. London: GL Assessment Limited.

It felt very difficult, encouraging people through an assessment. One of them was a sex offender who'd not been sent to prison and was on a tagging order. What was really interesting about that was he seemed really good at communication, but then when you did the CELF, you realised there were certain [weak] areas. That was such an interesting case because he seemed so articulate until you actually started assessing him. And you saw such a clear pattern of behaviour when he knew that he didn't know things. That was probably the most interesting language case I think I've ever had, because if I'd just met him I wouldn't assume [he had] any issue. He knew but he masked it, he knew exactly what he was and wasn't good at. So when we explained the task in the CELF, his demeanour would change. So if you said, "You've got to complete a sentence" or "We're going to ask you to put the words together", he'd be like, "Oh, I don't want to" and he'd change the subject and start talking about something else. **Keira**

Early intervention

Many key government policy documents highlight the importance of early identification and intervention with young people who are deemed to be 'at risk' of offending. The HM Government Youth Crime Action Plan (YCAP) (HM Government, 2008) cites supporting young people and their families and improving strategies for prevention of crime as two of the key aims. Youth offending teams play a critical role in meeting these targets and the YCAP specifically recommended that provisions for young people with SLCN should be developed further. Two of the students were involved in early intervention on their placements. The service that Callum joined had a specific remit to provide early intervention for children from the age of 4 years as they start their education. Although he worked directly with a small number of children, the remit was primarily met through training staff in the education and justice sectors. Callum described how the children were identified as being 'at risk' given their young age.

They do assessments…they work on early intervention so they identify children at risk, which tend to be brothers and sisters of kids who are already known to the [youth offending] service. I did an assessment on a boy…two of his siblings were already known to the service, another was known to the service as a victim not as an instigator. He was 9 but his language level [age equivalent] was 5. He was in line with development [delayed as opposed to disordered language development], but they identified him and they were trying to avoid the gap [between age and language level] getting bigger. **Callum**

Julia also worked with young people identified by the YOT as 'at risk', though her clients tended to be older.

We did some youth prevention work, so [with] people who hadn't offended. They started about 8 years old, but mostly the people were maybe 13 to 18. It was mostly based on the family and whether siblings had committed crimes… and the area they lived in…but the prevention work was usually because older siblings had been involved in the service. And behavioural referrals from school if people had gone into pupil referral units or had anger management issues. **Julia**

Intervention

The RCSLT has released a 'dossier of evidence' (RCSLT, 2012) which outlines the recommendations regarding speech, language and communication in the youth justice system, in terms of both training others and direct intervention. The report highlights work carried out by the Derbyshire YOTs, who recommended a 'three tier approach' to providing intervention within the youth justice system (Heritage, Virag, & McCuaig, 2011). In the first tier, they advocated the training of all staff working with young offenders to increase awareness and understanding of SLCN. The second tier recommended more in-depth training for core staff and the third for SLTs to provide direct intervention. The work carried out by the three students on placement encompassed all of these tiers, indicating the progress being made in delivering a more appropriate service for young people.

Training other professionals within the youth justice sector

Most staff within the youth justice sector have not received any training about identifying and working effectively with young people who present with speech, language and communication difficulties (Nacro, 2011). Most of the small number of SLTs who specialise in working with the youth offending population are involved in training others about SLCN to increase awareness and early identification so that the most appropriate support can be offered to young people within the justice system.

Callum primarily worked on the content of training packages for different groups of professionals, and then attended the training, which was delivered by his clinical educator. He helped to run sessions for the police force, Appropriate Adults, staff in pupil referral units, a school for children with emotional and behavioural disorders and primary schools. Callum found that a lack of knowledge about SLCN and the possible range of impacts was the biggest challenge that he faced. Much of the training offered was focused on educating people about how to adjust their own language to aid the comprehension of young people.

> We did training with a couple of primary schools on language levels. It was how to use language...rather than using complicated language, it's simplifying your words, slowing down when you're talking...it's making them more aware. We showed them clips of two boys who were quite eloquent in the way they were speaking and then another lad who couldn't explain why he was there [at a crime scene]. We were saying, "This is what we're talking about." **Callum**

Julia also worked with staff in an education setting, training those who had regular contact with the children identified by the YOT as 'at risk' of offending. She felt that this helped to raise awareness of SLCN whilst being a time-effective measure for a service with limited capacity in terms of speech and language therapists.

> A lot of the assessments were carried out in schools, then we'd do a lot of work with teaching assistants and SENCOs because they were delivering the therapy. The services weren't there to give regular therapy, so it was

all programmes and strategies. I think it worked in that given the limited resources, you saw the clients, their needs were identified, and then if they had significant needs you referred them on to a community therapist. Otherwise they had strategies in school for learning new vocabulary and memory. People were more aware of their needs. There wasn't really the scope for long-term planning, because people [clients] were only with the youth offending service for a short time. **Julia**

Julia and her CE also delivered training about SLCN to other members of the YOT so that they were more able to accurately identify children under their care who required assessment. This links with the recommended second tier of intervention, which advocates more advanced training for core members of within the youth justice sector (Heritage et al., 2011).

We delivered training to the youth offending team so if they thought, "I don't think he's [the client] quite picking up on what I'm saying", then they made referrals [to the speech and language therapist]. It was quite consultative. They did have quite a strong awareness [about SLCN]…not so much in the court. The magistrates apparently had training on language, the fact that a lot of offenders have language needs and they should tailor language in a certain way. But I went to court one morning and observed and it wasn't like that. Everything's technical and legal terms. **Julia**

All of the students visited a court to gain an insight into the legal system and the language used in this context. Like Julia, Callum also felt that the high-level language used was likely to present quite a challenge for young people with SLCN.

I was in court for a day, which was very interesting. I was having a look at the language levels. I wanted to see the process of what these kids go through, but it was looking at the language levels used by the magistrate, used by the legal clerk, used by the judges and it was very, very interesting. You could tell that these kids have no level of understanding. One magistrate had a referral order for this boy and he was going to do consequential thinking. Now if you said consequential thinking to somebody who has a learning age or a functioning age of 11 or 12, they don't understand. **Callum**

Although none of the students played an active role in any element of the legal proceedings, they did gain an insight into the role of their clinical educators with some cases that were going to court.

She would write a pre-sentencing report that would talk about assessment [results] and then how that impacted on his functioning and his consequential thinking if it was relevant to the case. She would basically be objective and say this is where the downfalls are and these are the consequences. **Julia**

Keira's clinical educator was also asked to give an opinion about particular clients that they had been working with both in the community and in a secure setting. These examples illustrate the wide scope of the SLT role within the youth justice setting.

My clinical educator had to write papers that were going to be involved in court cases. There was a boy who had been arrested and they queried him having autistic spectrum disorder. [My CE] had to go and see him and then had to write a statement for court about his view. My CE did it, as a student I didn't have responsibility for that…but my CE would often ask me my opinion. **Keira**

Direct intervention

Keira was the only student who delivered a notable amount of direct therapy during the course of her placement, primarily within the YOI setting. Due to the constraints of the YOI and the transient nature of the environment, the key challenge was the limitations in terms of how much contact Keira was able to have with her clients. This made it difficult to set long-term goals regarding therapy and meant that Keira needed to take a more short-term, reactive approach to her sessions.

The boys' days were very structured, so we would only be able to see them in the morning during what would be their education time, or pull them out in the afternoon during their education time. So you were very limited [in terms of] how much access you could have to them. A lot of the boys were in there for a short space of time, so you'd come across somebody who you'd really want to work with and then they'd go to court and be out, so it's quite a quick turnaround. You've got other boys who are in and out of the system the whole time. For people who are serving long sentences, it was basically prepping them for going up to adult prison, so that was a strange feeling. It was like prepping a child for going to secondary school... "This is going to be a different system and you're not going to have as much support". **Keira**

The evidence suggests that many young offenders with SLCN are disadvantaged in terms of accessing rehabilitation, educational courses and treatment because of their language impairments. Programmes that address anger management, healthcare and many within other areas are primarily delivered via spoken and written materials, but research suggests that approximately 40% of young offenders are unable to take advantage these programmes because of their communication difficulties (Bryan, 2004). Keira worked with professionals from a range of other disciplines with the YOI to deliver training programmes that were more accessible for clients with SLCN.

We did parenting classes with the boys, alongside the nurses. We would do things about how you can play with a child, the language and words they might use...so that it was an actual course that was run for the boys who were young fathers. That was really good, because that became part of their education...they got certificates at the end of it. The majority of them were all really positive towards it and they loved talking about their kids...they'd all kind of change when they started talking about their kids. **Keira**

In addition to running groups, Keira also worked one-to-one with some clients, in line with the third tier of recommendations for service delivery (Heritage et al., 2011).

It was a matter of making them [the clients] aware [of their SLCN], and also trying to figure out why they offend. People who had language difficulties would be like, "I just get really angry when people don't understand me and I just flip", then you're like, "Right, OK, so do you know why you're getting angry, what can you do, or how can you tell people?" So it was a lot of preventative stuff, just to try and help them not reoffend. There was one boy we ended up doing a lot about anger management basically...doing visual diagrams for him to mark how angry he was getting, then talking about the areas of his life that were making him angry. So it was gauging how much he understood about his behaviour. You'd start doing something to do with communication but then his anger became the issue so you'd kind of have to manage the task at hand. **Keira**

Summary

Although only a relatively small number of students were interviewed about their placements with young offenders, their experiences illustrate the complexities of working with young offenders. All of the students specifically requested their placements due to an interest in the client group that was sparked by their own reading and lectures at university, and so it is perhaps unsurprising that they all felt they had a positive experience. The students felt strongly that their enjoyment came from working with adolescent clients with speech language and communication needs. The fact that their clients were 'young offenders' quickly became incidental to the work that they were doing.

I do think it's about respect and respecting that person as an individual and forgetting what they've done for the time being, as long as they're not an immediate threat. So it was more just like adolescent language work but happened to be in that setting. **Keira**

Top tips from students

- Read up on the justice system and the common terminology, e.g., remand, tagging orders. These are very common terms so it is useful to have a real understanding of what they mean for the client.

- There are many different members of staff within a youth offending team, so try to read about the different roles and what they involve.

- Read up about the different types of rehabilitation methods used in the criminal justice system, e.g., referral orders, Intensive Supervision and Surveillance Programme (ISSP).

- Leave any prejudices at the door!

- Find out what is 'in' and popular with young people so that you can create age-appropriate resources based on relevant interests.

- Read the evidence-base about the links between speech, language and communication disorders and youth offending.

- Make sure that you interact with young clients in a manner that helps them to engage and relate to you.

Top tips from clinical educators

- Ensure that you have a good understanding of confidentiality because the post crosses boundaries across youth justice, social care, education and health and you may work with people from all of these sectors.

- Be prepared for things to not always go to plan. This is a client group that is difficult to engage with tasks so be ready to think on your feet. We also do not know who is going to offend, thus the work can be unpredictable.

- Have a good understanding of formal and informal language assessments

- Read up on the links between behaviour and speech, language and communication needs.

- MDT working is quite different to what you may experience on other placements. Do some background reading on youth offending teams and the demographics of the particular area you are going to be working in. This should help you gain a picture of the young people that you may encounter.

- Be aware that many staff in the youth justice service do not know as much as you about communication

- Give every client as much time as they need to answer your questions.

- Keep your language clear, simple, concise and to the point.

- Don't be afraid to use objects, photographs or drawings to support work in sessions.

- Always ask the clients if they understand what you have just said. If they say "Yes", ask them to explain it back to you. If they say "No", then it is up to you to explain again as many times as needed.

- Keep it simple. It is easier to make things harder for a client if you have pitched things incorrectly than it is if you have gone in at a level that is too difficult.

9 Adults with learning disabilities

Learning disabilities are lifelong conditions caused by damage to the brain before, during or after birth. The RCSLT (2009) states that although not an illness, learning disabilities are often co-morbid with physical, psychological and psychiatric conditions and range in severity. Learning disabilities have a lasting effect on development and are characterised by a limited ability to acquire new skills or information and impaired social functioning (Department of Health, 1998). Approximately 90% of individuals with a learning disability present with some degree of communication impairment (Bradshaw, 2007) and 80% of people with severe learning disabilities do not develop effective communication skills (RCSLT, 2006). A subgroup of people with learning disabilities present with 'profound and multiple learning disabilities' (PMLD) and display the most complex and severe types of impairments, often communicating only via eye gaze, facial expression or other nonverbal cues. Dysphagia is also common among adults with learning difficulties and can have a significant impact on quality of life (RCSLT, 2010). One third of all speech and language therapy provision in the UK is devoted to both adults and children with learning disabilities (RCSLT, 2006) and it is estimated that 0.46% of the adult population in England access services for people with learning disabilities (RCSLT, 2010). Challenging behaviour, such as aggression or sexually inappropriate behaviour, is more common amongst this client group, thought to be due to a lack of alternative modes of communication or self-expression (Enderby et al., 2009f).

Much of the speech and language-based intervention with adults who have a learning disability is based on the Means, Reasons and Opportunities model (Money, 2002), a paradigm that has roots in the social model of disability. The model focuses on enabling a client to understand others and express themselves, to have autonomous reasons to communicate and to be provided with opportunities for interaction. Communication strategies must be functional and appropriate to the context of the individual client.

In this chapter, six students recount their experiences from a range of placements with adults who have a learning disability. They describe the environment in which they worked with their clients, which ranged from community settings and colleges to forensic inpatient services. The students reveal the huge range of clients they worked with, and the assessment and therapy that they designed and implemented during their diverse range of placements.

Setting

The students saw their clients in a number of very different settings, illustrating the variety of provision and service delivery models for adults with a learning disability (ALD). Beth and Sue were located in a central office base which housed the MDT offices. They both visited clients out in the community: at home, nursing homes and day centres. Sara, Josie and Maria all spent their placements at sixth form colleges with tailored provision for adults with learning disabilities, two of which provided residential care in addition to education and therapies. Keeley experienced a rather more unusual environment, spending her placement working in a forensic ALD setting to support adults with a learning disability who had a history of offending behaviour.

Sue met her CE at the central office each morning, and they travelled out together to visit clients in a range of settings.

> It was community based, so going out from the office to see clients in their homes or community centres, either at home with family or in a house with other residents and a house manager and house staff. Lots of travelling. She [the CE] didn't see more than two clients in a day, I was really surprised, perhaps three at the most, but she did cover quite a big area. **Sue**

Beth had a similar experience in her community team but many of her visits involved carrying out joint sessions with other members of the MDT, most commonly psychologists, nurses or dieticians. She found that home visits could sometimes be a challenge.

> [It was] a real eye opener as to what you might find, you never knew what situation you were going to walk in on. I think it depended on the house because some you went into, they were very much like, "Oh come in, sit down", and then other places you felt like you were taking up their time, because they were not that keen for input. And that

was when it was a bit more difficult…you were trying to do what you needed to do and they had the TV on and were looking at their watch. **Beth**

Home visits also proved difficult on occasions for Sue, who visited a client with pica (the consumption of non-nutritive substances). Although her clinical educator had briefed Sue about the visit and the environment in which her client was living, she was shocked at the reality of her client's situation.

I did end up seeing one person who was [an adult with] pre-intentional, preverbal [communication] and that was a bit of a shocking experience from an emotional standpoint. My clinical educator warned me, just before we went in the house. It was really clinical…bare floors, bare walls, no curtains, a table and two plastic garden chairs, because she had pica and all sorts of difficulties to do with eating. Pica was quite common actually. So it was very, very clinical in there, not homely at all. It was quite shocking and she was really [at a] very early developmental stage. It was really shocking to see a grown adult, my age she was actually, to see an adult at that level developmentally. It's so incongruent as a first experience…the environment she was living in, the house, with two full-time carers around the clock. [The other residents] had to move out because of her difficulties. She couldn't live with anyone. So all of that, it is quite shocking when you see it for the first time I think. **Sue**

Keeley spent her placement working in a specialist forensic ALD service. There is evidence to suggest that adults with learning disabilities are more at risk than the general population of both committing crimes and being the victims of crime, and also that mental health conditions are more common within this client group (RCSLT, 2006). Consequently, there are a number of tailored services for this population and SLTs are often part of the multidisciplinary team involved in care and rehabilitation. Keeley had very little information about her placement prior to her first day and approached it with feelings of trepidation. However, she received high levels of support from her clinical educator and went on to develop a keen understanding of this specialist environment.

> It was classed as a hospital, but it was also classed as a prison, because the people there were sectioned under the Mental Health Act[19]. All of the people had some degree of a learning disability, the majority were mild, with a few with moderate [learning disabilities] and also many of them had mental health difficulties…the psychiatrists managed the treatment plans that each of them received. **Keeley**

The clients, both male and female, lived in small communal flats or houses with varying levels of security and were supported by a large multidisciplinary team of professionals. There were two specialist speech and language therapists who worked part-time at the secure hospital, spending the remainder of their time working with young offenders in a community setting. Keeley described the range of environments in which her clients lived and she visited to deliver her sessions.

> It was like any sort of mental hospital, because they were sectioned, they were there until the psychiatrist decided that they were well enough to leave. But it was meant to be quite a fast flow. People went into medium [security] and then they went to one of the lower houses with less security and were able to go out on trips. Then there were perimeter houses which were just outside the gates so they were almost back in the community and then there were the houses outside of the [hospital] in the community where the section was completely lifted. **Keeley**

Maria and Josie both spent their placements on sites that included specialist school and college facilities for children and adults with learning disabilities, but primarily worked with adults aged between 18 and 25 years old. Many of the colleges were residential, with students living in supported accommodation onsite. This allowed strategies to be implemented both in college and in the home setting. Josie worked as part of a large and diverse MDT at a residential sixth form college for adults with learning disabilities.

> There were two staff to one client. It was very specialised… the equipment, the facilities, a hydrotherapy pool…all of the classrooms had hoists. All of the LSAs (learning support

---

19 Mental Health Act, 2007

assistants) were very experienced, [there were] nurses, a medical centre. They had [clients with] dysphagia, so they had a whole kitchen for different food consistencies. They had a physio on site, an OT, an SLT...all in the same room. **Josie**

Sara also worked with her clients at a specialist college for ALD, but the students all came from the local area and most lived at home with their families. The college offered four different courses to students, who were allocated to a particular route based on a range of assessments and their medical diagnosis. Sara found that the setting required her to take a very flexible approach to planning sessions with her clients, but that the environment was conducive to this way of working.

Because it wasn't community based, you didn't have to go out and meet people...everyone was there. So if you didn't have chance to do a session...because they were always going out and doing other things, you hardly ever knew where people would be...you could just say, "It's fine I'll do it later", or "Once they've calmed down I could go and see them if they were ready to do some work". **Sara**

All of the students worked within a core mult-disciplinary team of physiotherapists, OTs, psychologists, dieticians, nurses and social workers. They all found that this gave them a much deeper understanding of the different professional roles and the boundaries between the related professions. Many of the students shared offices with people from a range of these disciplines and they regularly planned joint sessions to carry out with clients..

We were all sharing the office which was really good, because you got to just pick up on so much, which I hadn't had on any of my other placements. Those had been just speech therapists in the office or a one person office. It was really nice and people would chip in, especially when it was the assessment time. So the client would be assessed by everyone and then some people would say, "What was he like when you went to see him?" or, "He's very engaged, or very interested in working with me", and then somebody else would say "No, he didn't want to know, he didn't want

> to talk to us". So it was quite nice to get that, although you were seeing them on different days, you still got the feel for what they could be like in different situations, with different people. **Sara**

Maria took every opportunity that she could to understand the multidisciplinary environment, opting to observe physiotherapy and hydrotherapy sessions if her own SLT session had been cancelled. This afforded her the opportunity to observe the work of other professionals, but she also felt that she gained a more holistic understanding of her clients and the impacts of their communication difficulties in different situations. Sharing an office with other members of the MDT team meant that, even if the students had not directly observed another session, they were able to gain immediate feedback about their client's communication, which helped them to gain an understanding of whether their input was beginning to generalise to other environments.

> If you're working with someone intensely and then they go out for a day with OTs or teachers and they say "Ah [the client] used his communication aid to say this today" and you get that feedback…it is rewarding, you're getting somewhere and helping them. **Sara**

Josie found that the close working environment meant that she felt very well supported if she had a difficult session with a client and she felt able to discuss any issues with the wider team.

> There were days when you would come out of a session and think I'm useless, not only did that session not go right, I've no way of moving forward, I don't know how to do this. And the OT would say, "He's a really, really, really complex client, I don't know what to do with him either". Everybody was so sensitive and supportive in that way. **Josie**

Though the multidisciplinary environment proved a largely positive experience for the students, some struggled to understand the boundaries between the roles of different professionals. Josie found that she would often become involved in aspects of client care that she found interesting but fell outside of the speech and language therapy remit. As her placement progressed she began to understand these boundaries and learned when it was appropriate to refer clients on to other professionals on the team. Sara spent some time with the occupational therapist, hoping to learn more about her role and the links with speech and language therapy.

> I had a morning with the OT and she was explaining a lot about the switch work that she was doing and the cause and effect work. She was saying that a lot of the time in the community, that would be the speech therapist's role. And also with eating and drinking. The speech therapist said, "Once the spoon gets into the mouth that's my job, before that, getting it to the mouth...it's not my role." They have to distinguish, otherwise everybody could do a bit of everything and you don't know where you stand. **Sara**

Beth's experiences illustrate the importance of different professionals working together and having a sound understanding of each other's roles.

> There was some debate between the social worker and the speech therapist as to what is capacity...in a meeting I was in, the social worker had said someone didn't have capacity, whereas if [they had] adapted the resources they [the client] probably would have had capacity to make that decision. But because the social worker had given them the standard document, they weren't able to. **Beth**

Working closely in an MDT did mean that the students gained a much greater appreciation of the value of each of the different professions. Equally, they also found that speech and language therapy was a highly-valued discipline among their colleagues on placement.

> The psychologists did anger management and assertiveness courses. I had a chat with one of them and it was quite interesting because they said that it [speech and language therapy] was really important because they'd do a course with somebody and then realise that they'd not quite got the language levels to understand it. So everybody was tied in quite closely...there was an overlap between roles, but all the different professionals worked quite separately. **Keeley**

Due to the nature of the clients and the environments in which they were seen for speech and language therapy, all of the students found that they worked extensively with either keyworkers or care staff. This presented the students with a number of new challenges, but also demonstrated how vital it is to forge strong working relationships with those most familiar with the clients. Several of the students highlighted two key challenges. Firstly, they found that there was either a high turnover of staff or lack of continuity resulting from shift patterns that led to communication breakdowns. Keeley found that this was a particularly pertinent issue in the secure hospital, where incidents of challenging behaviour from clients often led to staff being moved around the facility.

> It was the carry over [of therapy] to staff that was quite difficult, and I think that was mainly because there was such a high staff turnaround. You'd go in and there'd be different people there all the time, so it was different from working with a family or a school. If something happened between one of the patients and the staff then they'd move. **Keeley**

Secondly, there was sometimes a perceived lack of support from some care staff for the intervention that the students wanted to put in place for a client. Many of Sue's clients lived in shared accommodation with several residential care staff who often differed in their opinions and their subsequent level of support for the strategies that Sue wanted to put in place.

> You [sometimes] felt the scepticism. There was definitely an agenda which was potentially very different to yours. The environment was a challenge, because all the other placements I've worked on, I've worked amongst other professionals, either allied health professionals or doctors who kind of talk the same language as you, you understand each other. When you're working in schools with teachers, you might not always agree the best way forward, or they may be sceptical about your therapy, but again, you feel like you're talking to somebody who is understanding your language. The really big challenge with ALD is dealing with the care system, that was difficult. You would get a real difference of opinion between the staff in a house sometimes. You might put something in and somebody thinks that's a good idea and somebody else is really sceptical. **Sue**

Despite the challenges highlighted by Sue and Keeley, Josie and Maria reported very positive experiences of working with care staff which aided their therapy and overall client care. Josie found that her client's learning support assistant (LSA) helped her to gain a better understanding of her client and the therapy that he had received in the past:

> I spoke with the LSA that had worked with the student since he was 4 and he was [now] 22. She was able to say when he really responded to a lavender smell, "I know why he's responding to that, his mother wears lavender". He really, really loved it. It was being able to appreciate that I could work with the client every day for six weeks and I will have a fraction of knowledge of that client. You need really good interpersonal skills...you've got to be sensitive to the fact that they know the client. You can't come in and say, "Oh, I have this brilliant scheme"...ask first what they've tried, so you don't come in with a brilliant idea and find out that that idea has been tried and for whatever reason it wasn't successful. They are the tool to get it to work right. **Josie**

Maria was initially nervous about the presence of her client's support worker in her therapy sessions, but she adjusted to the situation very quickly and soon realised the importance of his role.

> At first I was a bit like, "Oh no, what if I do something wrong?" But it was quite useful actually, because they know the clients inside out and most of them [the clients] are nonverbal so they had little things that they would do to indicate that they were tired, or maybe that they were going to have a seizure and I didn't know those things. So one of them [the support worker]...he was saying, "You might want to finish soon because it looks like he's heading for a seizure", so it was really useful having them there. **Maria**

Due to the potential for challenging behaviour in the secure hospital, Keeley carried out all of her therapy sessions with her clinical educator present. Despite initially feeling nervous about this scenario, Keeley actually found that she valued the support and this helped her to feel secure throughout her placement.

> In terms of safety, I always felt very safe with my clinical educator. There were a couple of incidents where some of the patients could be a bit inappropriate, but it was planned for and you were warned. My clinical educator was always with me, always with me. **Keeley**

Several of the students worked directly with their clients' families, both to gain information about their clients and to discuss therapy strategies which needed to be generalised over to the home environment. This presented a number of challenges which centred around the clients' capacity to make decisions despite their chronological age. Following her placement, Beth felt that she had come to understand how best to manage these complex situations.

> Respecting that the person is an adult and therefore needs to be treated like an adult, but that the family may still have that caring role. And knowing when you should be speaking directly with the client and when you need to involve the family as well. **Beth**

Maria had no direct contact with her clients' families because all of her clients lived away from home at the residential college. She found that she relied more on her clients' keyworkers to gain important information.

> It was difficult because most of them lived there. I only got to talk to them [the client's parents] on the phone, and some of them didn't really want to talk to me. It was difficult because you didn't get that face-to-face contact and the relationship with them. So writing reports to them and thinking 'I don't know really know you'…it was quite difficult in that sense. And there's their key workers, you sort of talked to them like they were the parents because they were with them all the time, they knew them…they were the ones you were getting most of the information from. **Maria**

Working in a community setting allowed Beth to have more direct contact with her clients' families during home visits. She was able to explain functional strategies to both the client and their families so that they could be implemented in the home environment.

I did home visits where families were present…in those situations you find yourself speaking more to the family, because they want to be kept in the loop, they're so keen to know what's going on and how they can help. And it might be a change that they need to make to the environment that'll impact upon the client you're actually seeing. I worked with a man who had a BMI [body mass index] of over 50 and the change needed to be made to his environment, and that was a joint visit with the dietician and involved a visual timetable, but obviously implemented by the family at meal times. So although he needed to be there, to see the visual timetable and to have it explained to him, it was more important that the family knew about it and how to use it. **Beth**

Caseload

Although all of the students worked with adults who have learning disabilities, their range of experiences highlights that this is an umbrella term which encompasses a wide array of clients with many different diagnoses and requirements. Sara, Josie and Maria were all placed in specialist colleges for adults ranging in age from their late teens to mid-twenties. All of the clients in Maria's setting had cerebral palsy, whereas Josie worked in a specialist facility for clients who had a sensory impairment in addition to other conditions. Research indicates that people with learning disabilities are between 8.5 and 200 times more likely to have a visual impairment and approximately 40% more likely have a hearing impairment compared to the general population (RCSLT, 2006):

I was working with adults with profound learning disabilities and sensory impairment, so they were often deaf, blind and autistic. There were physical difficulties, complex needs…massive, massive complex needs. So serious medical conditions, life-threatening medical conditions, dysphagia, cerebral palsy, migrating brain disorder. **Josie**

Sara worked with clients who had severe learning disabilities, many of whom were on the autistic spectrum. Depending upon their particular range of difficulties, the students joined one of four courses offered at the college. Most of the clients with ASD either joined the sensory or high-level ASD courses. There were also pre-entry and entry courses for clients with a range of cognitive abilities.

> Some had a year out between their special needs school and coming to college. But they all would have been in special needs schools before coming to college. Some students would be too anxious to [go to college] full time, so they might go for a morning. For some it depended on medication that they were taking. They might not be able to engage in sessions or within groups at certain times of day so might come later. Some take time off. If they're having difficulties they may not come to college for a month. **Sara**

Although Keeley did work with some older clients at the secure hospital, most were young adults. She worked with three clients regularly, and her experiences illustrate the variation among this client group, even within one very specialist setting.

> Their problems were so varied and there were no two people who were even remotely similar. I had three clients who I was seeing on a regular basis. One had a mild learning disability and SLI, very specific [difficulties] with morphology and syntax. And then another client who I was seeing, his learning disability was a result of epilepsy as a child. He had an almost a global type of aphasia as a result of his epilepsy. And I think he had head injuries as a child, I think he fell out of a tree. I found him quite difficult to work with…it was hard trying to find theory that I could relate to working with him, because he had so many different things going on. And there were also problems with his processing and conversations. Another client who I was working with on a regular basis had a very mild learning disability and showed some signs that you may see from somebody at the higher end of the autistic spectrum. So quite varied. **Keeley**

Sue and Beth both worked with adults from a wider age range on their community placements, but had regular clients with a comparable range of complex needs. Sue had one regular client with pre-intentional levels of communication and severe autism, and another who was verbal and presented with moderate learning difficulties. Beth worked with a gentleman who had only just been referred into speech and language therapy despite struggling to communicate for all of his life.

> [One of] my regular clients was an older man with learning difficulties who was completely unintelligible. It was his first referral to speech therapy aged 55, and nobody has understood him for 55 years. That was a massive eye opener. We realised people had really overestimated him, because he had never had a language assessment. You couldn't tell at all what he was saying and in fact he didn't have a reliable yes and no. He got referred for unintelligibility and obviously there was a much bigger problem. The original referral was because they were having issues with his understanding of money and paying for things at his day centre. He wasn't paying for things he needed to pay for. I think he had just been getting by with the level of support that he'd got. He lived at home, but he had live-in carers. **Beth**

In addition to enormous variability between different clients, many individual clients also showed huge fluctuations in their language abilities depending on a range of other factors. Many were taking medication that affected their attention and behaviour, something which had an impact on their ability to engage depending on the time of day their therapy session was scheduled. The students also found that learning difficulties were frequently accompanied by other factors such as visual impairment or anxiety.

> It was really challenging. Every client was so unique, so individual, because they had such an individual mixture of difficulties. Most of them had an element of autism, but then one client would be perhaps purely autistic, the next client would have visual difficulties as well, or hearing difficulties as well, or both. They'd have challenging behaviour. Every client was truly unique. You'd start thinking about their autism and how that was affecting their language and

> what you might put into place for them, but that was really
> complicated by their visual difficulties or by their cognitive
> difficulties. It just takes an awful lot more thinking about,
> and I think it's challenging. **Sue**

All of the students worked with clients who had complex medical needs, something which is more common in adults with learning disabilities when compared with the general population (Department of Health, 2004). This often proved to be a challenge in terms of managing therapy sessions and Maria found this the most testing aspect of her ALD placement.

> Most challenging was probably medical needs for all of the
> individuals there. [There was a] girl who was trying lots
> of different switches. Within ten minutes she'd be crying
> because she was in a standing frame in our session and she'd
> just be in loads of pain. And also getting her to move her
> head to the left, she found it quite difficult, but that was the
> only way we could know it was intentional communication,
> if she was moving to press her switch. A lot of them had
> seizures, so you always had their key worker with you. You
> always had someone with you because they were quite high
> risk medically. **Maria**

Several of the students found that they sought emotional support from their clinical educator, peers or university staff following a difficult day on placement. Many of their clients had a reduced life expectancy and presented with a range of complex medical needs and challenging behaviours. Sara reflected on her young female clients, feeling that their communication and cognitive impairments often led to a high degree of vulnerability. Maria felt that her clinical educators were very sensitive towards the potential emotional impacts of her placement, but found that she coped with this aspect more easily than she had anticipated.

> I was told at the beginning of placement that if you get
> upset it's fine, you can just go out of the room, don't worry
> we'll understand. But I actually managed it on placement
> better than I thought I would...I think it's probably because
> I thought, well what I'm doing is helping so that's fine and
> if they're giggling away at something then great, they're

enjoying it. And also 99% of them [the clients] didn't understand their own illness, so that made it easier. The illness was quite emotional, and them being the same age as me, some of them. And most of them were away from home. The girl I was working with only went home every four or five weeks for a weekend. **Maria**

Keeley also felt very well-supported by her clinical educator, particularly given the unfamiliar nature of the secure hospital environment. During the initial few weeks of her placement, Keeley's clinical educator took the decision not to discuss the offences that had led to individual clients being in the secure unit, so that Keeley was able to form opinions based only on her interactions with clients. During the later stages, there was some discussion about the clients' backgrounds and Keeley felt that this helped her to understand her clients better.

My clinical educator kept bringing it up, "How do you feel about this?" because there were a lot who were in [secure hospital] for sex offending. But I found it OK. I think I was just able to separate people's backgrounds from why I was there. I think it's knowing the boundaries. **Keeley**

Two of the students experienced clients passing away whilst they were on placement. In addition to dealing with the personal emotional impacts, part of Maria's role was to help other students at the college to understand the situation.

Whilst I was there, one client did pass away. They had a bereavement resource at the Trust and we went through it with some of the young adults. But it's whether they understand [about] this person being gone…have they gone because they passed away or have they gone away for a week? You don't really know how much they understood…it was quite difficult, but rewarding at the same time. **Maria**

Clients with challenging behaviour

All of the students regularly had therapy sessions with clients who presented with a wide range of challenging behaviours and initially found this a very daunting aspect of working with adults with learning disabilities. Challenging behaviour is often used as a communication tool by individuals who have language and communication difficulties (Chamberlain, Chung, & Jenner, 1993), and can take the form of self-harm, physical aggression and sexually inappropriate behaviour (Enderby et al., 2009f). Psychological and psychiatric diagnoses are also prevalent when compared with the general population (Enderby et al., 2009f). Sara found that liaising with her clients' support workers helped her to understand the best ways to deal with the challenging behaviour of individual clients and sometimes helped her to spot the signs that her clients were becoming agitated or distressed.

> I've worked with children with complex needs…they will grow up to become the adults that I was working with. But it was just completely different because they [the children] are so manageable and little, but then when you've got adults and they're barging around the corridors and you know, they've got this stubbornness and this assertiveness… you can't talk them round as easily as you can with little ones. Some [clients] need this sort of passive [approach], praising them, whereas others needed "You're doing this now". And it was hard to know. Because you wanted to be nice and you didn't want to order people around, but sometimes that was what they needed, and I think that I just expected that I would gauge that. But sometimes you just need someone who knows them to tell you "This is what they need". **Sara**

Prior to her community ALD placement, Sue's clinical educator sent her a summary report and asked her to prepare session plans for a client who she was going to be seeing twice a week throughout her placement. Unfortunately, Sue was only able to work with her client twice in total due to his unpredictable behavioural difficulties. Despite these challenges, Sue never felt that she was in a vulnerable position and had a very positive experience working with her client.

> He was in a real period of challenging behaviour, involvement of the police, attacking people. Staff had described how he was really affable, a really lovely person to be with, but he had some psychotic problems and he would just switch

and he'd become a completely different person. He was
fine in the sessions I had with him. I felt fine, because I was
there with a therapist and obviously they would have never
have had me in a room with him on my own. I probably
took it a bit too lightly because on the first session I had
with him, we were on a round table, I was beside him and
she [the CE] was directly opposite him on the other side
of this table. At one point I looked at her for guidance on
something and she just said, "Sit back a bit, sit back away
a bit." I probably wasn't aware enough of the danger and
she described to me after how she would always sit towards
the door side of the room so that if she needed to make an
escape, she could. But I felt fine about it, because I knew
that the staff wouldn't have let us go in if he was having a
bad day. **Sue**

Although the students were briefed in-depth about their clients prior to meeting
them, many still felt unprepared for how to deal with particularly challenging
situations if they were to arise during a session. One way that they addressed
this was by speaking to the learning support assistants or keyworkers who
knew the clients very well. Many of the clients were hugely variable in terms of
their behaviour and their ability to engage with sessions. The students working
in residential settings found that the environment enabled the flexibility
to reschedule sessions more easily than those who worked with clients in
the community. Sara found that her clients with sensory impairments were
particularly challenging in terms of their behaviour. She had some difficult
experiences during her placement, but did find that she was able to adjust and
deal with these challenging moments.

In the sensory group [there was] lots of challenging
behaviour...all sort of stimulatory things. There was one
student...you would constantly hear people say, "Put your
arms down, put your arms down" and you knew that was
the precursor to an explosion of this behaviour where he'd
just scratch his face, and then there would just be blood
everywhere. And I saw that in the corridor and I just
thought, I need to sit down and one of the physios came

in and had a chat with me. These are the students that you don't see out and about…they're supported all the time in different settings, so it was quite a shock to experience that…but you'd go in the next day and the student would be fine. So you think, "Well, it can't be that distressing for them", although it was quite distressing for people around them. But then you become…not immune to it, but it dampens down a little bit, because you see it and you get used to it. **Sara**

Many of the students were particularly nervous about pitching their sessions at a level and in a style that was appropriate and expected this to be particularly difficult when engaging with clients of a similar age. However, the students all found that they were able to adapt very quickly and enjoyed the process of building rapport. Many found that they had mutual interests such as music or magazines and they were able to prepare materials that meant sessions were enjoyable for both them and their clients. Beth followed advice from her clinical educator and ensured that she always took an inclusive approach to interactions.

I would just say to go in and have a chat with them, like you would go in and have a chat with anybody, and then from that you can adapt within your first session. But, obviously to read clinical notes so that you know what you're going in to, to prepare a little bit. With people who are nonverbal and people with PMLD, a big thing that my CEs focused on is that when you're talking about them, you need to talk to them. So even if you know that they're not understanding all of your language, they still feel included in the conversation, and whether it's someone else that answers for them, you're still addressing the questions to that person. It can feel a little bit strange, but then with people who are nonverbal, sometimes they'll give you thumbs up and things whenever you say their name and that feels a bit more natural, because you're getting some kind of feedback, even if it's not related to what you're saying. You feel like they're still part of the conversation. **Beth**

Assessment

Most of the assessment carried out by the students on placement consisted of standard departmental language screens that were used to assess whether or not a client was taken onto the speech and language therapy caseload. Keeley discovered that every person entering the secure hospital was given a standard screen as part of the admissions process. They were then assessed in more depth at a later stage.

> They were in [hospital] for a few weeks until they settled down, and then speech and language therapists would go and assess each person's language. The psychologists also did a cognitive screen. **Keeley**

Despite working in a very different environment, Sara was also involved in screening potential clients. She visited local schools to assess young adults who were due to begin further education in order to gauge their suitability for the college and also to help decide which of the four college courses would be the most appropriate for the client. The students were reassessed once they had enrolled at the college to ensure that their abilities and requirements had not changed in the interim period. These informal assessments examined language, cognition and behaviour, and were accompanied with referral information from both the client's previous school and from their family.

Sue carried out informal assessments during her placement with adults in the community setting. She found that the assessments usually needed to be very tailored to the clients' abilities and often served a highly functional purpose. One such instance related to the assessment of pain that her client was experiencing, based on evidence that suggests communication impairment makes it more difficult for a client to describe pain or symptoms (National Patient Safety Agency, 2004).

> Doing formal assessments can be very difficult given the range of difficulties that people can have. It's like a really complex jigsaw with people and their range of difficulties. It's very difficult for me to say what I used commonly, because there was no common thing. We [Sue and her CE] assessed somebody's understanding of pain...we had time discussing that before we went in to see him, discussing the approach that we had put together. He also had issues

with passage of time, we were assessing that [pain] and his understanding of the passage of time, because there was a feeling that [they] might be linked to challenging behaviour. **Sue**

Sara found that although formal, published assessments were appropriate for some of her clients, she found it particularly challenging to adapt most formal language assessments for those clients with sensory impairments, so for them adopted a more informal approach.

Some students…cognitively they could do it [the formal assessment], but there'd be other difficulties like visual impairment or hearing impairment or something that prevented them from taking part which was quite challenging. We had lots of real objects, so it was recognition of them and function of them. And we came up with a couple of things to test prepositions. Some of the students would [be able to see] light and dark, so it was having different coloured paper and say put these things on the blue paper and these things on the red paper. Just trying to think about the assessments and what they're targeting and trying to change it. Just because you've got a visual impairment doesn't mean that you can't communicate. **Sara**

Beth and Sara were the only students who carried out formal assessments on a regular basis, most commonly using the Test for Reception of Grammar (Bishop, 2003) to assess language comprehension. Beth carried out an initial assessment with a 55-year-old gentleman using the Renfrew Action Picture Test (RAPT), which is designed to assess expressive language in children aged between 3 and 8 years old (Renfrew, 2003). Despite her initial reservations about whether this was appropriate, she gained useful assessment results and felt that her client was comfortable with the assessments that she carried out.

It involved a lot of assessment…I was the first person to see him…I saw him for 10 weeks, the first 8 weeks was assessment. We did the TROG and the RAPT and then just informal things. I think it [the RAPT] felt appropriate, because he was comfortable with it and because we said at the start, some of these pictures are a bit silly but we just need to do them. **Beth**

Some of the students were also involved in assessing clients to help decide which form of augmentative and alternative communication (AAC) would be the most suitable. This involved a thorough assessment of each client's motor, linguistic and cognitive skills and then bringing all of the results together to decide on the most appropriate intervention. Sue made three home visits to a client in her early 20s who had recently begun to use an Apple iPod touch™ as her communication aid. The sessions primarily focused on her client's use of the device so that any specific needs could be addressed in further sessions.

> She and her Mum [had been] very much involved in the need for a much smaller device. She had a much bigger, dedicated communication device and she hated it, it wasn't cool and she didn't want to take it to college...she was developmentally much younger than her age, but had totally age-appropriate interests and wanted to talk about boy bands with her mates at college. She had loads and loads of vocabulary and pictures on it [the Apple iPod touch ™] and the job was just to see how well she was using it strategically, how well she was switching it on or off operationally. No one had really looked at the linguistic side...how well was she using the different word classes, how well was she using negatives...I put a table together based on verbs, nouns, places, people and then I just used games...slips of paper face down... we would take turns to pick one and it had "Show me where pencil and paper are". **Sue**

Many of the adults with a range of learning disabilities presented with dysphagia in addition to their communication impairment. Although the students were unable to carry out any direct assessment or therapy due to their lack of training, many did have the opportunity to observe their clinical educator working with these clients. Keeley and Sue both accompanied their CE to mealtime observations and videofluoroscopy clinics and helped to explain the risks of aspiration pneumonia to clients

Intervention

All of the students had ample opportunities to carry out direct therapy with their clients as opposed to designing programmes for other people to carry out. Many of the students commented positively about the amount of direct therapy that they were able to plan and implement and cited this as one of the best aspects of their placement with adults with learning disabilities.

> I really loved it, the whole thing, because it wasn't what I was expecting at all. I got to do quite a lot of hands-on therapy, whereas I thought it might be more dysphagia. But I've been able to practise therapy with clients. **Beth**

In terms of planning therapy, Keeley found that setting goals with her clients was more difficult than usual because of the environment in which her clients were based and often the long-term nature of their stay in hospital.

> I think one of the main things that I found challenging was setting short- and long-term goals when somebody is going to be in there [secure hospital] for the foreseeable future, it was quite tricky. And when to close your duty of care with that person, when that's appropriate. Because of the learning disability, I think you could go on and on and on, trying to work on things. **Keeley**

Beth was the only student to become involved in safeguarding, defined by the Care Quality Commission (2013) as "protecting people's health, wellbeing and human rights, and enabling them to live free from harm, abuse and neglect". She attended several MDT meetings concerning a particular client who lived in a residential care home for adults with learning disabilities and felt that this aspect of her experience on placement was one of the most demanding.

> There were real concerns about medication being missed or giving him tablets when he was on stage two thickener…so I went to a lot of meetings with care home managers and social workers and families about that. I found that quite difficult. Knowing that you had to leave and it was going to carry on, and that you were leaving someone in that place, where you knew they weren't being looked after properly and that they were unable to stand up for themselves. That was difficult. **Beth**

Josie and Sue both carried out Intensive Interaction (Nind & Hewett, 1988, 1994) with some of their clients and felt that their therapy had very positive outcomes. Intensive Interaction is a method of teaching preverbal children and adults about the fundamental aspects of communication such as attention, eye contact, gesture and vocalisations. Because Intensive Interaction promotes physical contact with the client in many cases, both students often found it difficult to judge the fine line between remaining within professional boundaries whilst using the techniques to encourage their clients to engage with the therapy. This is one aspect that they discussed with their CE; however, they were both overwhelmingly positive about the effects of this approach for the clients once they had sought guidance.

> Intensive Interaction was amazing, I was getting students to look at me, sustain eye contact…one girl, who I assumed didn't even know that I was in the room, not only reached for my hand, she held it. She had cerebral palsy with a startle reflex that was really sensitive. But if I did Intensive Interaction it would stop and she'd calm and she'd be able to just reach out and experience things she didn't normally experience. **Josie**

Functional therapy

A significant proportion of the therapy carried out by students was functional and often highly tailored to meet the needs of individual clients.

> We really put the emphasis on functional therapy or communication for the person and didn't get too bogged down in impairment. A lot of these people had been living with impairment for a long, long time and had found ways to get around it already. **Beth**

All the students really came to understand the importance of setting therapy goals that were meaningful to the individual and which would have a positive impact on their quality of life. In addition to very specific functional goals for particular clients, several students ran group sessions centred on activities of daily living or the development of social skills. Sara ran regular joint sessions with other members of the MDT for her higher functioning clients at the college.

> The higher level was mainly social skills and activities of daily living, so lots of cooking, gardening…lots of working

> together. We did lots of trips out with occupational therapists, going to shops, going to cafés…going shopping to get all the things they needed before their cookery class. So lots of things that would be able to be transferred once they finished college. That was the main focus of it, to [promote] independence. **Sara**

Sara also independently planned and ran regular group therapy sessions for some of the students at college with a diagnosis of ASD. Despite initially feeling daunted about this level of responsibility, she rose to the challenge with the support of her clinical educators.

> I think it was the idea of placement that was scary. When I called up first of all, I got an email to say "Can you set up a social skills group for ASD students?" And I was like, "Me?" So I had to set all that up, but it wasn't that bad. I had so much support and I think that's really important. **Sara**

Keeley worked regularly with an occupational therapist, carrying out group therapy sessions with residents of one of the bungalows on the secure hospital site. These sessions focused on functional and social skills, with goals such as planning a coffee morning event for their fellow residents. Many clients benefitted from the use of visual aids for support and several of the students spent time putting these in place for clients to support their day-to-day functioning.

> He [the client] didn't know when meals were finished, so would keep eating and eating and eating. So we were providing visual reinforcements [symbols] of "This is what you're having today" and then he took it off the board when he'd eaten it and then it was gone and that was it. So to help his understanding of when things were finished. **Beth**

Sue produced visual aids to assist her client's understanding of time, an aspect of processing that a number of her clients found difficult. She worked with him to produce a calendar of his significant events and appointments so that he could begin to understand the passage of time and plan ahead. Sue also worked with a client who was suspected to be in pain, but was not able to communicate this to others. Following assessment, she took a highly functional approach to helping her client communicate when he was unwell.

> We were trying to assess whether he felt pain, whether he had a concept of pain, because he had a lot of challenging behaviour and there was a suspicion that it may be linked to him not being able to tell people that he was in pain. So we wanted him to put it in [a] pain diary. **Sue**

Augmentative and alternative communication (AAC)

Perhaps the most common type of intervention carried out by the students was to implement augmentative and alternative communication (AAC) in a variety of forms. AAC systems are hugely diverse, but all are used to support or replace spoken language. The students gained experience of three types of AAC on their placements: signing, the Picture Exchange Communication System (PECS) (Frost & Bondy, 1994) and high-tech devices. Despite the high prevalence of communication disorders within the client group, research has shown that approximately 60% of people with learning disabilities do have the capacity to learn and use symbolic communication (The Foundation for People with Learning Disabilities, 2000). Three of the students were involved in supporting their clients to use the Makaton system of signing (Walker, 1978), either in place of speech or to support their expressive language, although none of them had any prior experience of Makaton other than the theoretical knowledge they had gained through lectures at university. Beth began her therapy by introducing Makaton to a gentleman who had never used it before. She learned the signs for his first 10 key words prior to her session, and then worked on these for a number of weeks with him, adding to both of their vocabularies gradually during the course of the therapy. Sara worked with a range of clients who had already begun to use Makaton, and so she took a basic training course prior to her placement and a more advanced course during her time at the college.

> My clinical educator said that I would need it [Makaton] and that she was running the second course [during] my placement if I was interested. So before that, I got onto the foundation course for two intensive days. I picked up quite a lot then and just found that because I was using it all the time, I picked it up quite quickly. I think it's amazing, I really do. I think it supports people so much. Even if they can do

one little sign for something that they can't say, they've just told you something that otherwise they wouldn't be able to [have done]. And for me, communicating with them, it's just that extra little prompt for them to think, "Oh that's the word or that's the symbol that I need." **Sara**

Maria also found that Makaton was a common form of communication on her placement at the residential college, although she was surprised at how inconsistently it was used by some members of the college staff despite the staff training that they had received. This is consistent with evidence from the RCLST, which states that carers and staff who work with adults with a learning disability may have low levels of awareness and training about communication (RCSLT, 2006).

I realised that even though [they had] done the training it doesn't mean it's always going to be used and I think that's quite difficult. Then on the last day it was actually a training day and we did a communication obstacle course for all the staff. All of them at the end said, "I do need to give them more time, I do need to listen to them", and most of them said, "If I know what they want, it saves me time not to ask them." One lady said she had been caring for someone for six years and only found out a couple of weeks ago that she loved milkshake and she said, "I've never offered her milkshake, because I know she likes blackcurrant." You actually need to push and say, "Maybe just do the Makaton sign there"…they know it, but obviously they've got all the medical needs on their mind and they've got to get them [the clients] to this appointment and that appointment. **Maria**

Sara worked with clients who used a range of AAC modalities on her placement and she was able to see how some of her clients might progress from one method of communication to another as their abilities and skills developed.

So the 'sensory students' start off [for] the first four months working on cause and effect and then you work up and you do switches, maybe move onto PECS. So there's all that low-

tech stuff, and then it moves up to the entry students who
are using very high-tech communication aids. **Sara**

The Picture Exchange Communication System (PECS) (Frost & Bondy, 1994)
described by Sara utilises symbols to encourage communication by the client
exchanging a symbolic picture for an item that they would like. This serves a
highly-functional purpose, encouraging clients to initiate communication and
gain more control over the choices that they make. High-tech communication
aids vary enormously, and all of the students worked regularly with clients
who made use of these devices. Maria and Sara initially experienced similar
challenges in finding a way to make communication feel natural when their
client was using a hi-tech communication aid. As their nerves decreased and
they became more familiar with their clients and communication styles, many
of these initial difficulties diminished.

> You had to wait a lot longer for communication, obviously.
> And it was hard to know when to jump in, because the girl
> I was working with, she had really good symbolic awareness
> but couldn't really read the words. So sometimes she'd get
> mixed up between symbols. And it was hard to know when
> to chip in and help her. And also when she asked for help, I
> always asked her if I could look at her communication aid,
> because it was a bit like, "That's your voice, I don't want
> to intrude". And looking at her, not at her communication
> aid. But I enjoyed it…as the placement went on it got easier
> as well, because I got to know them, so I knew when they
> were a bit stuck. **Maria**

Sue found AAC to be the most difficult aspect to prepare for in advance of
her placement. She found that until she knew the specific methods and modes
of AAC that her clients would be using, it was very difficult to know which
aspects to research. However, once her placement had begun, she did find it
useful to read more about the modalities and devices that she experienced and
found that her clinical educators were able to recommend useful resources to
further develop her understanding.

> I had done some reading around AAC, knowing that
> would be a big thing with people with learning disabilities,
> but it would be nice to [have done] a bit more. It's one of

those things... you'd like to do more, you'd like to be more prepared [but] until you see the clients you're working with you don't really know what preparation to do. **Sue**

Summary

The students were faced with a great number of challenges on these placements, owing largely to the additional complex needs of their clients and the environments in which they were seen for speech and language therapy. Despite this, all of the students faced the challenges head on, and gained a wealth of valuable transferable skills and specialist knowledge. The opportunities to deliver regular and frequent direct therapy enabled the students to put their theoretical knowledge into practice; something that all of the students felt they benefitted from greatly.

It was really, really rewarding...we can make a real difference. The steps are really, really small. Sometimes I've got frustrated on placements that we assess, assess, assess, discover what's wrong with them [the clients], identify a real need and then give it [the therapy programme] to the support assistant. But with these clients, you were with them [for] an hour. You'd have days where you'd make such phenomenal steps forward and the next week it's like that didn't happen. And my CE said, "It's such a long, long journey, we've got them from age 4 to 20 and our goal for [the clients at] 20 is picture exchange. So very small steps and a very long journey that you take with them." The days when it worked were just amazing, you know, so they made the bad days OK. **Josie**

Top tips from students

- Find out as much as possible from your clinical educator before your placement starts. Ask about the particular types of learning disabilities you are likely to experience, the range of severity and any likely types of challenging behaviours.

- Be prepared to think holistically about your client. Talk to other professionals involved in their care and take every opportunity to observe your client in a range of different situations.

- Prepare yourself for the emotional impacts of the placement. The clients can be very unwell and may be the same age as you, so it can be tough. Seek support from your clinical educator.

- The care environment can be very different from a medical or educational environment. When planning assessment and therapy, think about the client's environment and ensure that your ideas are suitable.

- Think about the client from a functional perspective. Most clients have a range of difficulties, so consider which are having the biggest impact on the client's quality of life and let this guide your therapy aims.

- Trust your instincts. If you feel uncomfortable, excuse yourself from the situation and keep yourself safe.

Top tips from clinical educators

- Read up about a range of conditions before your placement: autistic spectrum disorders, traumatic brain injury, cerebral palsy, visual impairment and hearing impairment.

- Research some relevant intervention approaches: Intensive Interaction, objects of reference, AAC, PECS, Makaton, social skills groups and total communication.

- Try to learn some basic Makaton signs before your placement.

- Read the *Valuing People Now Summary Report* (Department of Health, 2009).

- Develop an understanding of the Means, Reasons and Opportunities model (Money, 2002).
- Be ready and willing to initiate and respond to any attempts at conversation with clients and staff on the multidisciplinary team.
- Dress modestly, particularly when working with young service users or offenders.

10 Adults with acquired neurological impairments

Speech and language therapists work with a great range of clients who present with neurological conditions. Some work with clients who have neurological damage from birth, others with people who develop conditions through the course of life. Acquired neurological conditions arise following damage to the brain, spinal cord or peripheral nervous system, caused by either disease or injury. In this book, traumatic brain injury is considered separately because of the different demands and experiences of students who have worked with this client group on placement. The present chapter focuses on the experiences of students working with clients who have developed speech, language, communication or swallowing difficulties as a result of stroke or a progressive neurological condition.

Stroke is the most common cause of adult disability in the UK and causes a greater range of acquired impairments than any other condition (Adamson et al., 2004). Each year in England and Wales, 87,700 people experience a first stroke and a further 53,700 have a recurrent stroke (Carroll, 2001). Aphasia, motor speech disorders such as dysarthria and apraxia, and dysphagia are all common sequelae of stroke.

Stroke is the most common cause of aphasia, an acquired language disorder that usually results from damage to areas of the left hemisphere of the brain which control language function. Although there are no official figures citing the prevalence of aphasia, most studies suggest that approximately one-third of people who suffer a stroke will develop aphasia (Bakheit et al., 2007; Laska, Hellblom, Murray, Kahan, & Von Arbin, 2001; Petheram & Enderby, 2001; van der Gaag et al., 2005), and between 30–43% of these patients will have persistent, long-term aphasia (Bakheit et al., 2007; Kertesz & McCabe, 1977). There are no reliable data regarding the prevalence of motor speech disorders, though more than half of the clinical population is estimated to have dysarthria or apraxia of speech following sudden-onset neurological injuries such as stroke or head injury (RCSLT, 2006). Dysphagia is a swallowing disorder that can result from disruption to any of the four stages of normal swallowing. As many as 78% of people present with dysphagia during the immediate stages post-stroke (Martino et al., 2005) and, of those, 91% have a persistent swallowing disorder (Mann, Hankey, & Cameron, 1999).

Progressive neurological conditions may proceed quickly or gradually depending on the type of neurological damage associated with particular diseases. In the adult population, the most common progressive conditions with communication and swallowing symptoms are Parkinson's disease, multiple sclerosis (MS), dementia, motor neurone disease (MND) and Huntington's disease. Each condition is typified by a specific group of symptoms, though research has shown that between 30–80% of people diagnosed with a progressive neurological condition will develop significant swallowing and communication impairments (RCSLT, 2006).

Adults with acquired neurological conditions account for a significant proportion of the population who access speech and language therapy services. Almost every student in the UK will spend at least one of their clinical placements working with this client group, though in a variety of settings and often with a specific clinical focus. Because of this, nine students were interviewed about their experiences with this particular client group in order to gain a representative sample of the range of placements. Their accounts illustrate the range of settings in which clients may receive speech and language therapy: from acute wards and rehabilitation hospitals, to client homes and nursing homes in a community setting. The students worked with clients post-stroke and with those who were at a range of stages following their diagnosis of a progressive neurological condition. All of the students gained some experience of working with clients who had motor speech disorders, aphasia and dysphagia, though particular environments resulted in a bias towards particular speech and language diagnoses.

The setting

The range of student experiences reported in this chapter illustrates the breadth of settings in which adults with acquired communication disorders access speech and language therapy. Some of the students worked solely in an acute setting, operating as part of a multidisciplinary team that saw clients on a range of hospital wards. Other students worked with clients who had been discharged from the acute services into rehabilitation centres or hospitals. Community-based placements were also common, requiring students to make home visits or carry out their work in nursing or residential homes. In fact, many of the students spent time in all of these environments within one placement, enabling them to experience a wide range of clients and services and develop a host of clinical skills.

Working in an acute setting

Ella and Sophie were both based in acute hospital services for the duration of their placements, whereas Melissa and Danielle split their time between the acute and rehabilitation wards within a hospital. Danielle worked predominantly with clients who had suffered a stroke and had been admitted to hospital as inpatients.

> I was on a stroke ward which was the acute [ward] where they came in after going into A&E (accident and emergency). Then they [would go to] the rehab ward… it was a bit more long-term residence. And then there were a couple of [patients] that I did see on other wards… geriatric ward, general medicine… and that was mainly [for] swallowing. **Danielle**

The way in which acute speech and language therapy services are delivered varies across the UK. In many hospitals, the SLTs will have a caseload of clients who present with a broad range of acquired neurological conditions. In other services, particularly at larger hospitals, the provision is more specialist and some SLTs work solely with one subgroup of adult clients. This is illustrated by Sophie's experience where, despite working with adults with acquired neurological conditions, she had no involvement with clients who had experienced a stroke.

> I was in the hospital and it was acute, so we were based in an office and then the medical teams in the various wards would ring and refer patients. And it was mainly assessment, so it was people who had conditions like MS and Parkinson's [disease] whose swallow deteriorated, or a lot of people with COPD (chronic obstructive pulmonary disease). It wasn't stroke, because there was a separate stroke team, so it was everyone else…there were quite a lot of patients with dementia. **Sophie**

Students in the acute setting were all based in the hospital SLT department. On a typical day they met their CE at the office in the morning to review the list of new and existing referrals and then visited clients on the wards. During the afternoon, they split their time between more ward visits and spending time in the department writing case notes and planning sessions for the following day. Although all of the students enjoyed working with clients on the hospital wards, they highlighted several daily challenges associated with the environment. Protected mealtimes, visiting times and ward rounds took place at regular times each day, but were often unpredictable in terms of how long they lasted. There was usually a range of professionals involved in each patient's care and finding a suitable opportunity to work with clients often proved to be a challenge.

> So you might go and see a patient but then the curtains [would be] round…the doctor would be doing the ward round so all the people you wanted to see you couldn't see. So you would just have to wait. But that's just a part of it really, you know that they've got other priorities, it's acute so you know that you're not as important at that point. **Sophie**

Ella discovered that when she was able to see her clients, they were often not medically stable enough for assessment or therapy, or were not able to engage so soon after their stroke.

> Because they're in an acute stage still, a lot of them are very lethargic and you have a lot of difficulty trying to wake them up, which was actually, with a couple of our patients, the biggest challenge we faced. **Ella**

Many of the students based in the hospital setting had regular contact with their clients' families during visiting times. They were able to use these opportunities to learn more about particularly unwell clients from family members and this helped both in terms of gaining a more holistic sense of their client and in putting together communication books filled with personal information. The students also provided advice, information and strategies about communication and swallowing, but this was not always a straightforward process.

> Probably about a third of people had family members with them…obviously visiting times varied, so you didn't

always see family members. I found it quite hard, because it was such an emotional thing that people can't eat, or they have to have thickener in their drinks and soft diets. Some family members were sneaking in food and drinks. It wasn't really me that dealt with that situation. I just observed it so it wasn't particularly challenging to me, but it was trying to be polite and know the person's got the right...if they really want to eat then they will. But trying to explain to them how bad that is for them. **Sophie**

Some of the students actually found it more challenging to work with family members than the clients themselves.

I think in a way that was harder, because they [family members] were actively distressed and concerned about what was going on and [were] able to communicate that. When you were talking to them, trying to glean information from them, they were more concerned actually about when their husband or wife was going to get better...not really caring that you were there trying to make their time in hospital better because they didn't want them [to be] in hospital. **Ella**

Perhaps one of the most difficult aspects was trying to reassure a client's family whilst at the same time being honest and not creating unrealistic expectations in terms of language recovery. This was particularly so for those students working with clients who were in the very early stages post-stroke.

By the end of the placement I was confident to put my hand up and say, "I don't know, they might, they might not but we're doing everything we can to facilitate them to get better." I think that's definitely something that placement really helps you out on. **Ella**

Working in a multidisciplinary environment

All of the students functioned as part of an MDT, regardless of the setting; however, those based in hospitals had much more direct contact with the other team members. Some attended regular MDT meetings, others worked in specialist MDT clinics, and all worked with a range of staff on the hospital wards. Danielle attended weekly MDT meetings to discuss the patients currently on the ward. She was able to play an active role during the later stages of her placement, feeding back to the team about the status and progress of her clients in terms of their communication and swallowing. Ella also attended team meetings, and the information that she gleaned led to her adapting her practice to benefit of one of her clients.

> I went to one [MDT meeting] and fed back, which was interesting, because I saw how I could work alongside the physios and others. For example, I had a patient who worked better if she was sat up, so I tried to always go and see her after the physios had been and got her sat up. In that way we were able to collaborate together which was quite good. **Ella**

Most felt that their opinions were valued in these meetings, regardless of them being students, and their experiences illustrate the high regard in which speech and language therapists were considered within the MDT environment.

> It was good to chat to doctors and to see that they really valued the role [of a speech and language therapist]… the SLT talked about when she'd noticed something, for example vocal cord paralysis, and then she could say to the doctors, "This could be X" and that changed the medical team's thinking and contributed to a diagnosis. There were examples of degenerative diseases being diagnosed in that way. I really like neurology, so it would be so good to be able to do that…I didn't really think about being able to help diagnose at all [prior to placement]. **Sophie**

In addition to her usual role on the acute neurological wards, Melissa was able to spend some of her time at a highly specialist clinic for clients with motor neurone disease. There were two clinics, one for people with a new diagnosis and one for those who were in the later stages of disease progression. She explained her role during these sessions.

> It was mainly observational. I did a couple of initial assessments, just asking the general questions. But I was mainly observing the speech therapist and the dietician and

then I followed a man who'd just had his diagnosis to all of his appointments...the social worker, GP, physiotherapist, OT. It was interesting to be able to talk to him about how he felt about it and how his wife felt about it. I think it felt for them like a lot of information to have all at once...and all the practical side of it which I hadn't really considered, all the money [financial implications], the fact that he was going to have to finish work...that was all the social worker's role. And the physio had lots of information for him. I think because they'd just had their diagnosis, it felt like a massive amount of information. **Melissa**

The students in acute settings all worked with nurses, doctors and healthcare assistants on a daily basis. Although this was almost exclusively a positive experience, Ashley questioned whether her advice was sometimes disregarded because she was a student and was concerned about the impacts of this on the clients.

Working with the nursing staff on the wards...we'd give them recommendations for dysphagia and they were ignoring the recommendations that we'd set them. Or it got confused somehow... so I was having to keep reminding them. I guess it was quite hard because I was just a student, so they might not have respected my decisions like they would an actual qualified working therapist. It was quite hard. **Ashley**

Ashley did find that, as she became more familiar to the ward staff over the course of her placement, her opinions were valued and advice was followed much more frequently. Despite the raft of challenges, the students were very enthusiastic about their experiences working as part of an MDT in the acute setting and felt that the busy environment made every day different.

I liked working in hospital...the fact that you've got lots of different people around you is really good. **Ella**

Working in a rehabilitation setting

Once patients have reached a medically stable point in their recovery, those who require further high levels of care are often transferred to a rehabilitation ward. Patients may stay in this environment for a short time period, or the ward may offer long-term care to those who require interventions or monitoring that would not be possible in the community. Ashley spent some of her time visiting clients at home and in care homes and the rest of her week working on a neurological rehabilitation ward. She had spent her previous placement working with the same client group in an acute setting, and reflected on the different demands of these contrasting environments.

> If I compare this placement to another one...I worked in a hospital on the acute stroke ward, and that was hard because you see patients at the worst stages and they are very ill and that's hard seeing them like that. But I think it's quite nice seeing them in a community setting, because they're at home, in their own environments, and they are making lots of improvements and recovering, so it was nice to see that. It wasn't quite so difficult in that situation, but on a ward or rehab unit it was quite different. **Ashley**

Ashley found that client referrals from the staff based on the rehabilitation ward were frequently made without sufficient information and she found it a challenge to manage a constantly changing caseload on placement.

> We would often get requests from the ward within the hospital, asking us to pop up on the ward just to see somebody. And it wasn't an actual referral, it was just a note that we'd got written down somewhere. It was difficult trying to explain to them...I can't just pop up, with a full caseload, and they wouldn't give you any extra details about this client, you'd have to just wander up and just take what you got really. That was quite challenging having to explain to them [that they] needed to make a proper referral was quite challenging. **Ashley**

Five of the students worked in the community for at least part of their clinical placement. Most were based in a community health clinic, using this as their central location for meetings and administrative activities but spending most of their days visiting clients at home or in a range of residential care settings. Due to the nature of home visits, many of the students spent a great deal of time travelling with their clinical educator across the area covered by the service.

There was a lot of travelling so it was difficult getting up early, early mornings and travelling about an hour and a half some days just to get to placement and then doing a whole day. It was exhausting…you're having to spend a whole day with your therapist and having to try and be as enthusiastic as possible. Sometimes you're just exhausted…It was a wide area we had to cover, so it did seem the majority of the time was spent in the car rather than carrying out therapy, but that's one of those things about working in a rural area. **Ashley**

One of the key themes to arise from the students' discussions was their feelings about visiting clients in their own homes. Whilst most students acknowledged that their clients were more relaxed in their home environment compared with being in hospital, some students felt uncomfortable working in another person's home, particularly during the early stages of their placements or if several people were present.

One day, I saw this lady, she was in her bed in her son's house, TV in there, very small room, lots of photos of her grandchildren at the end of her bed. It was quite hard because then the community matron came in and the son and his partner were popping in and my CE was doing a swallow assessment. I thought, "Gosh, I want to stay out of the way." And when she was on her own then, when everyone was in the kitchen, I could chat to her then, she was lovely and we had a lovely chat. Sometimes I thought I was just going to crowd people and I should stay out the way. **Maya**

As the students built rapport and began to take on a more active as opposed to observational role, most felt that working with clients' in their own homes was a positive experience for all involved.

It felt quite strange going into someone's home but it was all right. It's quite nice for them because I think they feel more comfortable with someone going into their home rather than them having to come out, especially if their mobility's not so good. And especially after you've seen

> them a few times, you can talk about the flowers outside
> their house and get to know them a bit better, which is
> lovely... When I was just observing I always felt like I
> was a bit of a spare part, especially when their house isn't
> massive and you're all a bit cramped. I stood in the corner
> just watching. But as I started doing more of the therapy
> and more of the assessment, I felt fine, because I was there
> to do something. **Melissa**

Some of the students felt that it could be difficult to strike an appropriate
balance between maintaining a professional attitude and working in such an
informal environment. Some felt that building rapport with their clients was
a more gradual process as a result of the home setting and that it could be
challenging to make recommendations to clients.

> It was quite weird because you were going in with your
> professional head, but you're in someone's own home. There
> shouldn't be a power relationship, but you definitely might
> not feel as comfortable to say things that you'd like because
> you are in someone's own space. **Ella**

One of the other factors associated with home visits, cited by several of the
students, was working with family members. Ashley spent part of each home
visit liaising with family members or support workers, providing advice and
strategies about communication and swallowing. Although she was initially
nervous about this aspect of her role, she became more comfortable with this
over the course of her placement. Richard also worked closely with his clients'
spouses, discovering the vast range in terms of how involved they chose to
be in therapy. Some spouses left the room during sessions and returned at
the end for Richard to feed back on the session and explain carry-over work
to practise between sessions. Others were more heavily involved and these
sessions were usually more difficult to manage.

> I met J's husband...he was very, very supportive, very willing.
> She had only had a stroke recently...within a few months.
> Most of the time during the sessions he would be there.
> He joined in quite a lot with sessions, and wasn't always
> helpful...it made J feel under pressure and it wasn't giving
> me a full view of what she could do. He only wanted her to

do well…but the times when he wasn't there, she actually did better. And I think it was just because she didn't feel under pressure to do very well and she just did as she could. I didn't want to upset him, I didn't want to upset her. He didn't think he was doing anything bad. **Richard**

Several of the students regularly visited clients in residential or care home settings and initially found this a daunting prospect due to their unfamiliarity with the environment.

I hadn't been in many nursing homes. I'd been maybe to see elderly relatives, but I didn't know much about the workings and the routines and things. You see them [the clients] in the lounge and there's lots of distractions going on. I had to see one gentleman who was quite advanced with his Parkinson's and his voice was really, really quiet, really soft, and the TV was blaring out and the nurses are going past going "What do you want to drink?" and I couldn't hear, and I had to lean in [to say], "Sorry, I didn't quite catch that.". He was quite dyskinesic on one day as well and I nearly got hit. So, yes, that was an experience. I said to this gentleman, "Are you OK here or shall we go back to your room?" But you couldn't move him, so you just had to see them where they were. **Maya**

Richard was particularly concerned about the level of care that his clients were accessing and was keen to find out more about the care homes from his clinical educator prior to the initial visits. He observed high levels of care at the homes he visited and felt that he got to know his clients better as a result of working with them in their own environment.

I always asked [my CE] before I went to the home…there were three residential homes that I went to…I always liked to know if it was a decent one, because I don't like the idea of people not living somewhere comfortable or not having their needs met, or not having somebody to speak to. In fact, they were all very nice. The staff were really nice. I think it would have just prepared me more than anything. I wouldn't have changed how I behaved, but it was just nice to be prepared for how it would be. **Richard**

A number of the students joined their clinical educators in providing dysphagia management for clients in nursing homes. Ashley visited a number of her clients in homes that catered specifically for people with dementia.

> There were a few nursing homes…it mainly was dysphagia that we did there. It was seeing clients with dementia, doing swallow assessments, things like that. I was quite lucky, I didn't see any complicated cases. It was giving the staff the support really and saying they are doing the right thing, giving them the reassurance. **Ashley**

Will also worked with many clients who had been diagnosed with different types of dementia and were in the middle-to-late stages of disease progression. He developed a keen interest in dysphagia management as a result of his placement, and worked closely with the care home staff to provide information and advice about dysphagia and the associated risks. He was particularly shocked to find that some of the staff had very limited training about dysphagia, so providing information was a critical part of his role in these settings.

> The naivety [of some care staff] about the medical side of things and the impact of a swallowing problem was a real shock. I think, in hospitals, nursing staff have had lots more training about dysphagia. I think the nursing home carers and staff often have less…in one home I went into they'd had no training at all. I'd given them some advice…"No biscuits, soft diet only, please be really careful, she needs full supervision, she has got dementia and she's leaving a biscuit in her mouth and I'm really worried that these crumbs are going to go down the wrong way". We had left the room, gone to see somebody else, come back and the lady was chewing on a biscuit. That really hit me. Although I'd explained, because the training isn't there, the information I'm passing on isn't going to be grounded on a good basis of understanding. The information I'm giving is kind of going over their heads…not because they don't care…they just haven't had that training and that's not their fault. As we left, the manager came and spoke to me and I was saying to her, "I have passed it on, but I don't think it has got through to the people who were giving the

lady the biscuit." It was really good to see that being able to explain the consequences prompted the new manager to say, "I'd really like some training for my staff." I think recognising that your role is to educate is actually really important. **Will**

Caseload

Some of the students worked predominantly with clients who had experienced a stroke. Those who were working in an acute setting found that many of their clients were still very medically unstable and this presented challenges in terms of finding appropriate times to work on their communication and swallowing. Most of the students had a varied caseload that included some clients with post-stroke aphasia and dysphagia, and adults with progressive neurological conditions. Many of the students felt extremely nervous during the early stages of their placement, particularly if they had not worked with an adult client group on previous placements. Research has shown that this is very typical, and despite the theoretical training provided by all qualifying speech and language therapy programmes, most students have little confidence about communicating with adults who have aphasia and report high levels of anxiety prior to these placements (Finch et al., 2013).

> I was initially nervous, it was daunting, I hadn't really worked closely with adults. I think my level of comfort varied [depending on] how poorly they were, or what kind of condition they had. The first week I met a lady with Huntington's disease…and of course from lectures I knew all about it, but actually seeing the person with it…it was tough. There were lots of people in her home and it was quite a small room and I remember there was a dietician there, there was me and my clinical educator, there was the lady on the sofa and her husband was walking in and out of the kitchen because they were doing the thickener for her food. I was sat there observing and thinking, "Gosh, this is completely new and I feel out of my depth." And then, from that extreme, to somebody who's maybe had a mild stroke, or an early stage of Parkinson's, where they're not

actually too bad and they're still intelligible, they can still crack jokes. **Maya**

Like all of the students, Richard did lots of research prior to his placement, but was still initially very nervous about remembering all of the information and about building rapport through conversation with adults who had communication impairments.

> I went in feeling absolutely terrified...I was trying to read everything I could possibly read. I was nervous about using the cognitive neuropsychological model[20]...which actually didn't really come up. I was nervous about trying to remember everything to do with MND, MS and aphasia. I feel very comfortable going into a room with a child and knowing that I can get them on side almost immediately. And although I'd had some experience working with adult clients, I was still nervous about just having conversation. But I'm glad she (CE) didn't say, "Wait until next week, you just observe this week." I'm glad I was thrown in and just did it, 'cause I would only have been terrified the next week and the next week after that. **Richard**

The wide range of medical conditions inevitably led to clients presenting with an array of speech, language, communication and swallowing difficulties. Several of the students with a varied caseload found the experience valuable, but felt that they were less able to gain a depth of knowledge about their clients and their conditions. Conversely, the students who worked predominantly with clients post-stroke felt that they gained valuable knowledge and experience of this client group, but perhaps were left with a narrow perspective in terms of working with adults with acquired neurological disorders.

> There was head injury, stroke patients, a lot of dysarthria, dysphagia and a few [people with] Parkinson's, MND and MS. It was a big range which was really good. I guess I only saw a snapshot of each thing...I wasn't able to get into the nitty gritty of it all, I didn't feel as though I gained a lot of new knowledge about the diagnosis. **Ashley**

---

20 Patterson, K. & Shewell, C. (1987). Speak and spell: Dissociations and word-class effects. In M. Coltheart, R. Job & G. Sartori (Eds), *The Cognitive Neuropsychology of Language*. Hillsdale, NJ: Lawrence Erlbaum

Many of the students reflected on the variation in severity of symptoms that they observed amongst clients with the same medical condition. Working with clients at different stages, either in disease progression or recovery from stroke, proved difficult for several of the students who found it difficult to know what to expect when they were visiting new clients. Those working with clients who had progressive conditions began to understand the likely prognosis for their clients who were at an early stage in their disease progression. Many of the student accounts suggest that they found it particularly emotionally challenging to work with clients diagnosed with motor neurone disease (MND). There are several subtypes of MND which lead to different symptoms depending on the involvement of upper and/or lower motor neurones. However, all of the subtypes are characterised by a progressive decline in motor function, which can affect speech, walking, swallowing and respiration and the decline in function can occur rapidly in many patients.

> It was the varying levels of severity for me I think at the different stages [of disease progression]. There was one lady with MND who was nonverbal and she wrote everything down. It was quite tough...her husband wanted to speak for her all the time...and she wanted to write it down herself. She was a very, very independent and strong-minded lady. Then I saw someone else with MND. He was in a wheelchair and I think his wife had dementia and looked quite emaciated. The house had been converted and he came down in the lift. He was anarthic and he had a litewriter, he was really, really unintelligible. I saw quite a lot of variation of Parkinson's. There was one gentleman who had no tremors but it was just his speech, and he was so motivated and focused...he was on the waiting list for 'Loud' [Lee Silverman Voice Treatment™], and he was like, "Oh yes, I really want to do this, I really want to focus on my speech." He was still quite young and it was early on in his diagnosis and I knew he'd go for it. But then, one [client] in a nursing home and another one I saw as well, you knew that you couldn't do much more for them. **Maya**

In contrast, Melissa felt that she gained little experience of the range of symptom severity described by many of the other students as she worked primarily with clients who she felt did not present with severe communication impairments.

> There wasn't anyone where their "Yes" and "No" were
> inconsistent. Quite a few of the patients [were] 90% fine.
> It was just the last few bits that we were tweaking. I think
> because of the caseload, the fact that it was so small, I was
> given anyone that wasn't too complicated. **Melissa**

Despite working with a varied group of clients, the students observed that many of the same skills were required regardless of the client's specific presentation.

> It wasn't as different as I thought it would be actually.
> Because, obviously, for all of them you have to make sure
> your communication is nice and clear and make sure they
> understood everything. **Melissa**

Several students discussed the complexity of the clients that they worked with on their placements. One of the challenges was in understanding the interaction of different impairments to gain an insight into the client's functioning.

> You don't often get patients with purely a swallowing
> problem, they're almost bound to have the communication
> stuff, alongside cognitive impairment. In Parkinson's disease,
> you might get somebody who's also got dementia alongside
> that, and then there's cognitive dysfunction, so it is much
> more complicated. **Will**

The psychosocial impacts of their clients' communication and swallowing difficulties had a significant impact on the way in which students related to their clients and all the students found that they needed to be sensitive and tuned into their clients' emotional status. They all felt that they gained an understanding of the enormous changes to quality of life that neurological conditions can cause for both the client and their family and friends. Richard reflected on the sudden and unpredictable nature of stroke and the devastating impacts that can change a person's life in an instant.

> A 63-year-old lady I was working with who now lives
> in a residential home had quite a severe stroke and she
> was completely physically impaired and wasn't able to
> do anything for herself. [She had] limited speech, better

understanding and better in conversation than in assessment. But also showing signs of depression, of how her life used to be. She's not ever going to be able to leave the home, I don't think…[She was] looking after her grandchildren every night, cooking tea, taking them swimming and running a garden centre as well [before her stroke]. Massive, massive change, and her husband was really struggling as well. It was very sad. **Richard**

Richard also worked with a number of clients who had been diagnosed with a progressive neurological condition. In these cases, his clients were coming to terms with a diagnosis, experiencing the gradual onset of worsening symptoms and usually had a very clear understanding of their likely prognosis. These circumstances brought with them a different set of emotions and difficulties for his clients.

I met a few people with motor neurone disease. But only in the early stages. One man that I met, he was having problems with speech and with eating. He wasn't up for a PEG[21] at all. And he was a retired pharmacist so he knew the implications of it all, which was a bit sad. He'd been to all of the medical meetings, he'd done all the research and he knew what the situation was and got a little bit upset. And his biggest problem was the social impact, because he liked going for dinner with his friends, he liked people coming over, he liked going for a drink, and he struggled on the phone when he spoke to his daughter, because she didn't always understand what he was saying and that's what upset him. **Richard**

Building rapport

The ease with which the students built rapport with their clients varied depending on a number of factors: the age of the client, the number of sessions, and the emotional stability of their client. The students had a varied caseload in terms of the ages of their clients, with the youngest often in their 20s and the eldest

---

21 PEG: percutaneous endoscopic gastrostomy. This procedure allows nutrition, fluids and medication to be delivered directly into the stomach.

clients in their 90s. Many of the students found it particularly emotionally demanding to work with clients who were of similar age to themselves but, at the same time, discovered that they were able to build strong working relationships with such clients.

> I used to see a client who was around the same age as I am, so she was perhaps 24. I think working with someone who was around my age and [wanting to] do the same sort of things as me, that was particularly hard, seeing her difficulties, that was hard. We did have a really good rapport, and we got on well together, and I think she enjoyed having me rather than perhaps an older therapist. She felt comfortable working with me, which was nice. I could relate to her. **Ashley**

One of the primary concerns held by many students prior to their placements related to building rapport with elderly clients. Some were concerned that they might have little in common with their clients, whereas others were particularly worried about directing sessions and giving advice to clients who were significantly older then themselves. However these concerns dissipated as they began to form working relationships.

> It felt less weird than I thought it would. I think especially as a final year student, I felt like I knew my stuff a bit more. I think if I'd done it in my first year it would have felt like, "I can't tell these people what to do, they're older than me." But now I feel all right with it, especially having built a relationship with the ones that I saw every week. **Melissa**

Many of the students were extremely nervous about meeting their clients for the first time, and were concerned that they would find it difficult to make conversation without the aid of the sorts of activities that they were accustomed to using with paediatric clients. Richard found that his nerves reduced as he got to know his client and the sessions had a more specific purpose.

> The first man that I worked with, his only difficulty was really apraxia, and he was the first client that I met. It kind of got easier from there because he was very articulate and he liked conversation. He was knowledgeable, I learned

something every single week, and he was a chatty old man, so that was useful to break me in. But even then I remember sitting, and she (the CE) said, "I'm going to do the assessment but do you want to do the conversation part first?" So I obviously said, "Yes", but didn't want to. And I remember…I couldn't think of anything, I couldn't have a normal conversation, so I just left it then up to [the therapist]. I just felt it was staged, I hadn't met him before, and you're relying completely on yourself having a conversation, rather than a puzzle or a book or a game. But after that it only got better and better. By the second week I felt fine, apart from that it was therapy the next week, so obviously there was that panic about being observed during therapy, but by the third week I felt comfortable. He was a really, really nice man so I felt fine with him. **Richard**

Relationships between the students and their clients were also strengthened by the progress made by clients over the course of therapy. The students were able to observe the positive effects of their therapy and found this a highly rewarding aspect of their placement.

Working with aphasic patients, I think that's what I enjoyed most of all. It's nice to see progression. I worked with one chap quite closely, and at the start he was very impaired. I had about ten sessions with him and I saw such a big improvement. It was just lovely to see that. I was able to see the same clients over the weeks and was able to develop a strong relationship with them and in the end I was going off to do visits by myself. It's nice to do that, because it's less pressure when you're working one on one with a client and there's not a therapist watching over you and I think it's a way of finding your own style of doing things really. And I was able to feed back after the session to the therapist, you felt like it was a proper job really, how it would be in a real life, you know, the real world. **Ashley**

Melissa worked with clients who not only demonstrated recovery but were also able to recognise the improvement in their own skills and report back on the impacts of these changes on their lives.

> One [client] came back every week and he was like, "I feel so much better, this is amazing, thank you so much for your help.. And with a couple of the ones that I saw every week, they would turn to me and say, "What do you think?" rather than talking to my clinical educator. **Melissa**

One of the challenges faced by many of the students was dealing with the emotions of their clients during sessions. Emotional lability is a common consequence of neurological conditions and many clients were also still coming to terms with the long-term impacts of their diagnosis. Many of Sophie's clients had a relatively new diagnosis of a progressive neurological condition, and she found it particularly challenging to build new relationships with these clients.

> I found that really hard, with some people it was fine, but others…the way they [the therapists] spoke to the patients, bearing in mind they were ill, they were talking about watching TV, and part of my feedback was "You should just chitchat", and I felt like I didn't want to chitchat. They were really ill, they were really upset, I didn't know what to say. **Sophie**

It was not only general conversation that challenged the students. Several found it very difficult to judge when to end a task or a session if their client was upset. Richard found that he was able to learn from his clinical educator about how to manage these kinds of difficult situations.

> She [the client] varied every week in her mood…she was never rude or unpleasant to be with, it's just that she was often a little bit upset, or if she found things difficult, she'd get upset. So I would say, "Are you finding this difficult? If you want, we can leave it there for today" because I was scared I was really upsetting her. But then [my CE] would say, "Well, it is a bit difficult but it's meant to be difficult, so if we try one more thing and you still struggle we can stop." Because I didn't want to see her upset and I didn't want to upset her, I immediately stopped, but once [the therapist] had shown me how to do that I put it into the next few weeks. **Richard**

Ethical decisions

Several of the students were surprised by the scope of ethical decisions that they and their clinical educators were involved in making, particularly with clients who presented with dementia or dysphagia. In her work with adults with progressive neurological conditions, Sophie regularly attended MDT meetings to discuss the ethical issues associated with clients who were not complying with feeding and swallowing recommendations. Although she did not necessarily play an active role in these meetings, she learned a great deal from the discussions and decisions that her clinical educator was involved in making and gained an insight into this aspect of the SLT role.

> There were more ethical decisions, not necessarily mine, but you really had to think about the ethics of things like PEGs, and I hadn't really thought about that before. There was a lady who kept pulling out her NG tube, she really didn't want it, she wanted to eat and drink, so it was, "Do you let her eat and drink…she's at the end of her life." It was trying to work out what was in her best interest really. If they're really adamant [the client], the medical team make a decision to eat and drink at risk, knowing that they might aspirate and then try and give them advice on avoiding it. **Sophie**

Will worked predominantly in nursing homes that offered care specifically for people with dementia. He found that consent and capacity were issues that he dealt with on a regular basis and that the situations could be particularly complex if a client was in a residential care environment.

> Patients with dementia are just so complex, and the fact that a lot of these people have been deemed to not have the mental capacity to make their own decisions…similar to the way with children where you've got the parents as the guardians…in nursing homes you're double checking with the nursing staff, the carers, family members. I found that quite hard because I think these are individuals who've obviously got their own minds and decisions, but on a piece of paper it says they haven't got the capacity to make an informed choice about something. So I think it

is a shock. When you're filling in a form about whether or not they've given consent, and could they follow your oro-motor instructions, it is harder, and you've got a lot more factors to consider. Whereas a patient who has had a stroke is able to communicate through pictures and gesture or has a carer who is closely involved. I think it is harder within a nursing home when you're not necessarily seeing the patient's family, you're working through carers. **Will**

Assessment

Client assessment formed a significant part of all the students' placements and most carried out a combination of formal and informal assessments. The students working with clients during the acute phase post-stroke spent much of their time administering initial screening assessments to gain a baseline score and direct further assessment and intervention. Danielle found that her clients spent an average of five days on the acute stroke ward before either being moved onto a rehabilitation ward or discharged home to recuperate in their own environment.

> We did the FAST[22] and then we did a departmental screen and the Mount Wilga[23] as well if that was deemed suitable, but we [started with] the FAST. It was useful, it gave you an overview. We did a lot of informal [assessment] through conversation as well. So you have a chat with them first and then you go in with a screen if necessary. I did find with a couple, from the informal conversation you could suss out what was going on with a client. **Danielle**

The initial screen was either followed up with further in-depth assessment of particular areas of difficulty, or Danielle would provide her clients with short-term communication strategies such as writing or a communication book.

---

22   Enderby, P., Wood, V., & Wade, D. (2006). *Frenchay Aphasia Screening Test (FAST)* (Second edition). New Jersey, US: Wiley-Blackwell.

23   Christie, J., Clark, W., & Mortenson, L. (1986). *Mount Wilga High Level Language Test*. Sydney: Mount Wilga Rehabilitation Centre.

Sometimes we did the Boston Naming[24] or the TROG[25] for receptive and expressive [language]. And then reading and writing…the reading was either single words or we were encouraging them to read newspapers. Writing… predominantly people were right handed. We'd tell them that we couldn't do a massive amount at that stage. It's just waiting to [see if they] got the feeling back, and if not then working on compensatory [strategies], but it tended to be in the community that we did that. **Danielle**

Ella also worked with clients post-stroke, and was surprised at the variation in aphasia severity, even during the acute stages post-onset.

In the acute setting I was working with clients over the age of about 65, who had come in with strokes [and] were normally 2 or 3 days post admission. A lot of them I did standardised assessments with, like the Frenchay Aphasia Screening Test or the Frenchay Dysarthria Assessment[26] and I also did the Apraxia Battery for Adults[27]. And a couple of informal assessments, to test reliability of "Yes/ No" response. There was one woman who was completely globally aphasic who had no output whatsoever, and I had other people who I'd go and see and there was literally nothing wrong with them whatsoever once we'd gone through an assessment. It was literally the occasional word [finding difficulty]. **Ella**

The students on a split placement across acute and community services gained an insight into the differences between assessment procedure in these settings. Some found that there was more time and flexibility in terms of assessing

24   Kaplan, E., Goodglass, H., & Weintraub, S. (1983). *Boston Naming Test (BNT)*. Philadelphia: Lea & Febiger.

25   Bishop, D. (2003). *Test for Reception of Grammar - 2*. Oxford: Pearson Assessment.

26   Enderby, P. & Palmer, R. (2008). *Frenchay Dysarthria Assessment (FDA-2)* (Second edition). Austin, TX: PRO-ED.

27   Dabul, B. (2000). *Apraxia Battery for Adults (ABA-2)* (Second edition). Austin, TX: PRO-ED.

clients away from the acute environment and preferred this aspect of their placement as a result.

> With the rehabilitation, you got stuck into it, that was better for me. I preferred that part of the placement. I couldn't do acute all the time, because it felt a bit like a production line. Even though I liked it, you're doing the same thing. **Danielle**

Despite Maya and Melissa both working in community settings, their experiences show the range of approaches to assessment taken across different services. Melissa predominantly used standardised assessments to measure her clients' level of functioning and found that familiarising herself with the tests prior to her sessions helped her to administer them without difficulty.

> I did lots of formal [assessment], I did lots of the CAT[28], lots of bits of PALPA[29], Boston Naming…I did some dysarthria assessments as well, [the] Robertson[30] and Frenchay (Dysarthria Assessment). I'd done none of them before 'cause I'd never had an adult placement before. [They were] quite self-explanatory. Once I'd done them a few times, I felt much more comfortable with them. They were all quite self-explanatory and as long as you had a look through them before, they were all fine. **Melissa**

Maya used a small number of formal assessments with most of her clients, but predominantly took a more informal approach to assessing her clients' level of functioning and devised many of her own materials during the course of her placement.

> Looking back, I thought I'd do lots of formal assessments and I didn't. I used the CAT, and I did the short Boston Naming. But it was informal assessment really and everything was functional. I devised my own case history and screen. **Maya**

---

28 Swinburn, K., Porter, G., & Howard, D. (2004). *Comprehensive Aphasia Test (CAT)*. Hove, East Sussex: Psychology Press.

29 Kay, J., Coltheart, M., & Lesser, R. (1992). *Psycholinguistic Assessments of Language Processing in Aphasia (PALPA)*. Hove, East Sussex: Psychology Press.

30 Robertson, S.J. (1982). *Robertson Dysarthria Profile*. London: Robertson.

Intervention

The amount and type of therapy carried out by the students varied enormously and was closely associated with the environment in which they were seeing their clients. The students based on acute hospital wards reported that they carried out very little direct intervention other than providing their clients, families and ward staff with short-term communication strategies and advice. In most cases, patients spent only a short period of time on the acute wards before subsequently being moved to a rehabilitation setting. This was an unexpected aspect of placement for those students, who found that they saw a high number of patients for initial case history and assessment sessions, but had little continued contact in the days and weeks that followed.

> I thought we'd do more therapy. We didn't do any. Even in that setting [acute neurological ward], I thought we'd do some. But it wasn't like that really. **Sophie**

Students based on the rehabilitation wards or out in the community had the opportunity to carry out much more intervention with their clients. Some took a purely impairment-based approach to therapy, whereas others carried out functional therapy more frequently. They worked with clients who had a range of diagnoses, but most commonly their therapy was for clients with aphasia, motor speech disorders and dysphagia. Richard's experiences not only show the range of clients on an adult community caseload, but also the need for a flexible and individualised approach to planning intervention.

> One had a stroke and he had some comprehension and word-finding difficulties initially, but the main problem was verbal dyspraxia so we were working on that and he was doing very well. Then another lady that I was working with also had a stroke, [she had] complete understanding but some cognitive difficulties, so memory problems. We started off doing word-finding strategies but because of her memory, it wasn't really that effective. So we referred her for a conversation partner or for a stroke group. She said that was better for her, because it [meant she wasn't] sitting on her own. Through no fault of the people that worked there, [in the nursing home] she didn't have any social interaction and it was just because they were so busy doing everything else. **Richard**

Many of the students gained experience of impairment-based and functional therapies and also worked regularly with other members of the MDT to meet common therapy aims.

> For dysarthria it was doing breath support and intonation mainly. Obviously breath support is the foundation for everything, so we did lots of that. Then with communication patients [post-] stroke, I had one lady who couldn't tell the time, so I was involved in that, which I didn't really expect. And then I did a joint session with the OT to do writing with her, because that was another thing she really wanted to do. So those things I hadn't really expected that would be my role really. Lots of letter sorting, anagrams, quite a bit of semantics. It tended to be phonology and semantics… most of it was expressive. **Melissa**

The students who were able to work with clients regularly throughout their placement gained great satisfaction from helping their clients to progress and meet their therapy aims. They were also able to observe the differences in efficacy of therapy depending on the client, and began to realise that the same type of therapy is not always effective for clients who present with the same diagnosis.

> I did some of the 'Loud' (Lee Silverman Voice Treatment™) sessions, I really enjoyed that. It was tough at first because it wasn't like your conventional therapy. I felt like I was being really bossy and thought, "I'm being disrespectful here, 'cause I'm just saying loud, louder" and that's how I felt really. I enjoyed the theory, it's interesting the theory behind it. I saw one lady…I'd seen the videos from day one to the end, she'd come on so much, she was fantastic. But then another gentleman, he was on his second lot of Loud training (LSVT™) and he just hadn't calibrated, so he wasn't there. **Maya**

They also found that getting to know their clients over a period of time helped them to tailor their interaction and feedback to suit individual clients, making therapy a more effective and enjoyable process.

> I'd been doing word-finding things with her, but then we moved on to drawing and gesture because they were her

strengths, and then did naming after that. So once she was able to gesture, or once she had been able to draw it, then encouraging her to name it, and if she needed help, phonemic and semantic cues. But she was amazing and I just thought, "Do you know what, I'm going to do some quick naming with her and just see how she does", and she did it really well. It really helped if you're really upbeat with her and said how well she was doing. **Richard**

Ashley worked with one client in her 20s and took a purely functional approach to boosting conversational skills and social interaction. She used her early sessions to introduce and practise strategies, building her client's confidence before taking the sessions into a realistic scenario to encourage generalisation.

I liked the fact that we got to work in their own environment where they felt most comfortable, and you could work on a lot of functional communication skills. There was one person in particular, I loved it, it was with a young lady. We planned a session to meet in a coffee shop and we were working on her conversation skills and her ability to ask for a drink, something really simple like that was a massive challenge for her. So we were able to plan the session, did a little bit of role-play, and she knew what she had to say, and I met her there and stood with her and she did it by herself. It was great to see that and it was nice to work in a different environment. That was a brilliant thing to do. **Ashley**

Dysphagia

Dysphagia is a swallowing impairment, usually caused by neurological damage or illness. It can have major psychosocial consequences and seriously impact on a person's quality of life. It can also lead to aspiration pneumonia if food or drink are taken into the lungs. Clinical guidelines highlight the importance of rapid assessment and diagnosis, diet modification and multidisciplinary management of dysphagia (National Institute for Health and Care Excellence, 2008).

The students based in acute settings were not surprised to find that clients with dysphagia formed a significant part of their caseload, though they were not expecting to work with clients who had such a wide range of diagnoses. Melissa estimated that approximately one-third of her clients had post-stroke dysphagia, 50% had a diagnosis of Parkinson's disease and the remaining 20% were adults with a learning disability. This illustrates the enormous variety of clients that students may work with during just one placement. Several students found that they worked with elderly clients whose dysphagia had been discovered upon admission to hospital because of another problem with their health. In these cases, dysphagia was often detected by nursing staff who referred clients to speech and language therapy for a more thorough assessment and diagnosis. Ella found that she spent much of her time assessing clients who had developed dysphagia following a range of surgical procedures.

> It wasn't necessarily with the stroke patients, it was more out in surgical wards…people who'd come in for other things and then a swallowing problem had arisen. I had one woman who had been brought in to have a hip replacement and after her operation completely lost the ability to swallow. Possibly from being intubated, that was one thing we looked at, but I left not knowing [the cause]. **Ella**

The role of students in working with clients who present with dysphagia has been debated in the literature and addressed by policymakers for well over a decade. In 1999, the RCSLT published a set of guidelines that included recommendations for pre-registration dysphagia training on undergraduate and masters level qualifying programmes (RCSLT, 1999). The key implication was that qualifying courses needed to provide students with a basic level of theoretical knowledge and skills so that they could competently work with clients under the close supervision of an experienced speech and language therapist whilst on placement. The RCSLT is in the process of reissuing an update of these guidelines to reflect current practice.

Most of the students gained some experience of working with clients who had dysphagia on their adult placements, though their level of involvement varied significantly depending on their clinical educator, personal choice and the complexity of the clients. The RCSLT guidelines (RCSLT, 1999) are a set of recommendations rather than being prescriptive in nature and so, unsurprisingly, the students were afforded extremely variable levels of autonomy on their placements in terms of working with clients. Maya adopted a purely observational role, whereas Sophie and Ella were permitted to take on a slightly more active role towards the end of their placements.

> The majority was communication because that was the choice that I made. I did do dysphagia but obviously I'm not qualified to actually do anything. I felt the swallow, I did the basics with the dysphagia but nothing more than I'm allowed to do at my level. I was quite happy with that, I think it's such a responsibility. I actually quite like dysphagia but I didn't feel confident enough and there's so much to know about it. I saw three videofluoroscopy clinics, which was really good. And it was interesting because I could actually identify things after my second clinic. **Ella**

Although Sophie felt more comfortable in an observational role, she gradually became concerned about how the lack of practical experience would impact on the development of her clinical skills. This was something that she discussed with her clinical educator and she began to take on a more active role under close supervision.

> It wasn't too challenging, because of the nature of it, because you can't do anything yourself really. You can do a little bit of feeding and mixing drinks, but you aren't expected and you can't be expected to be independent. So there was a lot of observation. So I did things slowly and developed over the placement, I did a little bit more and a little bit more. So because of that gentle introduction, it wasn't that challenging really. I didn't know how I could possibly get a good grade, because I wasn't doing much at first. But as time went on I did more. **Sophie**

In stark contrast, Melissa was given much greater responsibility for managing her dysphagia caseload, though still closely supervised by her clinical educator.

> I did all of it basically. She (the CE) was there. But I did the initial assessment questionnaire and then I got to feed them and I got to palpate the swallow as well, it was amazing. Obviously she did it as well and we went through the dysphagia checklist afterwards and decided what we thought it was. I was a bit nervous at first because she kind

of chucked me in at the deep end, but it was really good and I was like, "Wow, I feel really confident and really happy." I'd done all the bits separately, but then it was just doing them altogether and then taking the lead a bit more. But after I'd done it I was like, "Brilliant, I want to do another one, great." I seemed to have quite a lot of autonomy on the placement which was amazing. **Melissa**

The students primarily saw clients for an initial assessment of their swallow and made dietary recommendations on the basis of their findings. For those students who were experiencing dysphagia for the first time, assessment initially proved challenging.

It felt a bit invasive at first, because obviously they're trying to eat or drink, and when it's patients that are a bit older, their posture's not so great. Trying to get your hand right in there to be able to feel [the swallow] felt really awful. But my clinical educator said, "They don't mind and you need to do it and they've probably had it done before." **Melissa**

Despite the somewhat repetitive nature of dysphagia assessments, all of the students felt that they were continually challenged by their clients and their range of needs.

The days were quite similar in some ways, but the patients weren't. So you always saw something completely different for every patient really. So there was that variety, but there was a lot of standing around, waiting to be able to see people's notes and see patients. **Sophie**

Many of the students were involved in the continual review of clients as their swallowing function improved or deteriorated. Despite working with clients who had progressive neurological conditions, Sophie was often still able to observe improvements in function as her clients recovered from acute episodes of illness.

You'd see them first of all, and then you'd review them, so if they were still there the next time I was on placement, we'd go and see them again. That was good because it helped me to see a bit of progression. Some of them might not have been on oral fluids, and then you'd assess them again when they were better, like if their COPD improved, then you could put them back on normal diet. **Sophie**

Sophie discovered that despite the fact a session may focus on dysphagia, her interaction skills were just as important as they were when working with clients on their communication. Clients with dementia made up a significant part of her caseload and her reflections illustrate the challenges of working with clients who have a complex set of symptoms.

You did need to use your communication skills, especially if they had dementia, but we didn't do any communication assessment or therapy at all, and we didn't really do any dysphagia therapy, it was literally just assessment and putting people on diets really. We did lots of bedside assessments. I did referrals to videofluoroscopy. They took place in the hospital on a day I wasn't there but they did show me the DVDs of the patients I'd seen, their videofluoroscopys, so that was really good. It was good to see…you thought somebody was aspirating from what you saw and observed, but it was good to get that confirmation. So [for clients with] dementia, it was things like trying to give instructions that they were able to understand, and asking them to follow instructions, and [helping them to] understand why they were not allowed to eat and drink. And you were explaining, but then ten minutes later they wanted a cup of tea and it was horrible to have to say "No" again and again. **Sophie**

Assessment of clients with dysphagia was not restricted to the acute setting, something that most of the students had not considered prior to their community-based placements.

It was mostly dysphagia, which I loved. But there was a lot of communication stuff that kind of came with the dysphagia as well, I suppose. It was probably 30% purely for communication, 70% for dysphagia. So it was quite heavy on the dysphagia [which] I wasn't expecting. I think it was really good because my only experience of dysphagia was in an acute setting and I just thought that was where a lot of it happened. **Will**

Will's placement in the community gave him an insight into the long-term impacts of dysphagia through his work with a range of clients at home and in nursing homes. He gained a much wider perspective on how recommendations made by therapists would be carried through into the home environment following discharge from hospital.

> I think that was the biggest thing for me…that all of the swallowing assessment protocol that we'd been taught was really helpful in terms of the theory, but I'd really only thought about it in the acute setting, in terms of a patient sat in bed with the nurse at hand. And actually, to go into somebody's home and have to be thinking about, "OK, what could they have to eat or to drink, who's involved, who feeds them, can they feed themselves"…it's all very different to the early acute stage of somebody that isn't responsive, can't open their mouth. There you're doing literally oral hygiene rather than a fully-on swallow assessment, so I think it was definitely really good to see the whole thing in practice. **Will**

Will realised that visiting clients in their own homes gave him a much deeper insight into the range of impacts that dysphagia can have on quality of life, and that he needed to consider his existing knowledge in terms of this very different context. These experiences also encouraged Will to reflect on his clients from a more holistic perspective and he consequently felt able to work more effectively and empathetically with clients who presented with dysphagia.

> I'd read about all the continuing problems that you get following a stroke or dementia in terms of swallowing, but to actually see people three or four years post-stroke, sometimes still having difficulties…to see people with a progressive disease taking hold and it worsening…it was really helpful to see the long-term consequences within their home, and I think that's the difference…when you're in a hospital you kind of think, "It's a patient, they come in, they stay, they go out." Whereas when you see them in their own home, it's very real, that actually this is somebody with a life, a family, having meal times. For me that was not unexpected, but just really helpful in terms of solidifying

that looking holistically at a patient is really important, seeing them in their home environment is crucial and that was really helpful. **Will**

The emotional impacts

The students all reflected on the emotional impacts of their placement and their reactions to working with clients who were unwell and going through a very difficult stage in their lives. As their placements progressed and the students formed relationships with their clients, they developed a much greater insight into the impacts of their clients' neurological conditions. Like many of the students, Ella tried to separate her personal reactions from her professional role and found this approach helped her to cope with difficult situations.

> It was quite upsetting sometimes, because you'd look at someone and you'd think, "Oh my gosh, you can't communicate back to me, you're stuck inside" and you can see that they're really, really trying...but then on the other hand, you see it as "Well, maybe I can do something to help this person, because without me it's going to be worse." **Ella**

Will's experiences echoed those of Ella. He worked extensively with clients diagnosed with progressive neurological conditions such as motor neurone disease, and found his clinical educator to be a great source of support and advice following difficult sessions with his clients.

> It's the fact that you're not just seeing a patient with a communication problem, you're not just seeing a patient with a swallowing difficulty, you're seeing somebody that has got a really complex medical background, and that's the thing that often has the biggest emotional impact, I think. Seeing somebody with MND at home, really deteriorating, even from one visit at the beginning of my placement and then another visit at the end...seeing such deterioration, it would be very easy to just sit and think, "Oh, this is really sad, I don't want to do this." My clinical educator was brilliant, we chatted about it and I think just

> taking the perspective of, "OK, what can I do to help", rather
> than, "OK, I'm going to sit here and get upset"… being very
> positive about it and actually seeing the fact that, even as a
> student, you've got a role to play in helping to enhance the
> quality of their life now, rather than debating and being in
> turmoil over where they're going to be in a year's time, I
> think it's really important to think, "What can I do now?"
> That's what made me deal with it better. **Will**

Students on peer placements were able to gain extra support from one another
and several of the students talked to academic staff within their university
department about particularly difficult episodes. However, all of the students
acknowledged that the most important source of support and advice was
their clinical educator and all emphasised the importance of forming a strong
working relationship.

> How do you prepare for it…it's very difficult to know, isn't
> it really. I'm not sure you can prepare for it. I suppose it
> depends very much on your personal circumstances, who
> you've got in the family who might be poorly with certain
> conditions that you might come across. I think the important
> thing is having a good clinical educator who will check that
> you're OK or [who] is open to you coming to them saying,
> "Oh gosh, I found that a bit difficult." **James**

Several of the students raised the issue of working with clients who had the
same conditions as their own family members. This posed a particular challenge
in terms of dealing with the emotional impacts of placement.

> In dysphagia I came across some situations which had
> personal relevance for me. My (relative) has Parkinson's and
> I saw a couple of particularly severe Parkinson's patients…
> you see the future potentially for your relative. And as much
> as it was good for me in that I got a picture of what might
> be coming, it was definitely a bit shocking. **James**

Melissa spent a regular part of her placement working as part of a multidisciplinary
team in a clinic for clients with a diagnosis of motor neurone disease. Like
many of the students who worked with clients with this diagnosis, she found
this to be the most demanding aspect of her placement. Melissa co-ran the

SLT consultations with her CE and reflected on a particularly difficult session attended by a gentleman with a very recent diagnosis of MND and his wife.

> Working with [clients who have] MND…I found it very emotionally draining, that side of it was really quite upsetting. Quite a few other people in the clinic at the time were a bit further along (in terms of disease progression), he was like, "That's going to happen to me and that's going to happen to me." So that was quite draining. I said, "Not necessarily, it doesn't happen like that for everyone." I think his wife was thinking much more about the future, whereas he was much more here and now, could only think about getting through the next week. And they were so young and their kids were younger than me. Yes, the MND clinic was definitely the hardest bit of the placement. **Melissa**

Working with clients who had neurodegenerative diseases proved the most difficult aspect of these placements for all of the students, and many found it difficult to reconcile the fact that they were working to help clients whose level of functioning was in a state of decline.

> Somebody with Parkinson's, they're deteriorating and they're looking at you, and they want you to say that it'll be OK, but you can't, so that was quite hard, I think. That was quite hard when it was degenerative and you knew that they probably weren't going to get better. **Sophie**

Despite these very real demands, the students all felt that they were able to make a positive contribution to the wellbeing of their clients and many found their experiences highly rewarding. Melissa reflected on some of the differences between working with adults and children and felt that working with adults often led to a greater sense of achievement for both herself and the clients because they usually had much greater awareness of their loss of function.

> You get the happy side of it…stroke patients making some real progress, and I thought, "Wow, actually I do make a difference." It's really, really incredibly rewarding, because if you think about it, adults have had communication and speech and suddenly it goes. So being able to get any of

> that back is so rewarding and it was a brilliant feeling for
> me, and it was a brilliant feeling for them. **Melissa**

The range of reactions to these placements appeared to depend partly on the nature of individual students. Danielle and Ella both found that they were able to separate their emotions from the work that they were doing with clients and felt that this helped them to provide care that was more objective for their clients. Maya found this more of a challenge and questioned her reactions.

> If you are a sensitive person it was quite hard sometimes.
> On maybe one or two occasions I went home feeling quite
> low, but I didn't break down or get upset in front of anyone.
> I often felt, "Gosh, they're so young, it can happen to
> anyone and what a terrible disease." I wondered if perhaps
> I'm a bit too caring, and it affected me too much, when in
> fact of course it's going to, I'd not seen anything like this
> before. **Maya**

One aspect that all of the students found difficult was knowing how to respond appropriately if clients became upset during sessions. They felt that lectures had prepared them as much as possible in this respect, but the reality of working with real clients in testing situations was something that could only be addressed through experience and this was sometimes a distressing experience for all concerned.

> I did [feel prepared] in terms of the theoretical teaching, but
> in terms of all the emotional stuff around it, I don't think
> anything can prepare you for that really. You can talk about
> it, but actually being in that situation is still completely
> different. I had a couple of stroke patients crying when they
> got frustrated. Being able to react to that appropriately…I
> don't think you can teach that. **Melissa**

Richard's experiences with a regular client who had post-stroke aphasia highlights the range of issues that clients often deal with in addition to their communication or swallowing impairments. Examples such as these illustrate the importance of students getting to know their clients and of being aware of the wider picture and the way in which specific difficulties fit into the context of an individual client's life.

The lady who used to look after her granddaughters... that was upsetting. She was just so lovely as well, and she had photos of before she'd had a stroke with her little granddaughter, and her physical appearance was massively different...she had lost a lot of weight. And she was in pain quite a lot, so a couple of times she'd be really quite upset and cry and it was because she was in a lot of pain. It was loads more emotional than any other placement I've been on. **Richard**

Although the students anticipated many of the challenges they faced, some were more unexpected. Will sought support from his clinical educator following a visit to one client in very difficult circumstances.

I think I went into feeling like it's inevitable that some of the things I was going to see were going to be emotional because it [placement] is a stressful environment. But really there were aspects that were unexpected shocks to me in the sense of how I reacted. One lady in particular that I met, she'd been in hospital nearly a year... she'd had a massive stroke but no nursing home would take her because she had continually had *C. difficile*[31]. She was on a PEG so her nutritional needs were being met, but nobody was communicating with her because she was pretty much nonverbal. I heard about this from a member of the nursing staff and I was stood there thinking, "Oh my word, I didn't know that was possible for anybody to have to end their life in the hospital with nothing on the walls of their own, none of their own bedding, pillows, pictures, just in a hospital room...and nobody knew how to communicate with her. **Will**

---

31   Clostridium difficile (C.diff) is a bacterial infection of the digestive system. Those most at risk of developing C. diff are people who are over 65 years old, have been treated with antibiotics, have an underlying medical condition and have been long-term residents in a hospital or other healthcare setting. Health Protection Agency. (2009). *Clostridium difficile Factsheet.*

Summary

Despite the difficult and sometimes emotional experiences, many of the students gained a great deal of satisfaction from forming relationships with their clients and many felt privileged to be part of a team that was supporting people through such a difficult stage of their lives. Ashley's comments about her last few days on placement echo those of many of the students, affirming the positive experiences of most students who embark on these challenging placements.

> Saying goodbye was hard. Especially towards the end of the placement, where it came to the last few sessions that I had with the patients…just 'cause I had worked with them so closely and it was difficult saying goodbye. A simple thing like that is hard, emotional. You'd have to be quite a hard person, I think, to not feel anything at all. **Ashley**

Top tips from students

- Be prepared for working in a hospital and working with some clients who are unwell. Thinking about how you might deal with situations beforehand may help you deal with emotions as they arise.

- If you are using a cognitive neuropsychological model, try to link each of the levels with specific tasks. This should make it easier to make decisions whilst on the ward and enable you to work with a range of clients.

- Try to do some reading after each day that relates to the real clients that you have seen. This will help you to understand the conditions and remember the information more easily.

- Be aware of the different types of aphasia but remember to treat your client as an individual, not just the label they are given.

- Be prepared for the positive and negative emotions that you may feel and don't be afraid to seek support either from your CE or academic staff at university.

- Ensure that your therapy is always functional and relevant to the client that you are working with.

- Prepare some conversation topics for an initial appointment. Family and travel always seem to be good icebreakers!

- Practise carrying out a bedside swallowing assessment on family and friends, this really helps to build confidence.

- Keep a notebook with a list of medical acronyms so that you can read all of the client's medical notes.

- Try to gain some experience talking to older people. All my experience had been with a paediatric caseload and speaking to adults is completely different. Make sure appropriate praise is given and also know when enough is enough for them, and be able to gauge that because some get tired very quickly.

Top tips from clinical educators

- Make sure that you understand what a stroke is, revise your neurology and have an awareness of the likely brain regions that may be affected.

- If possible, volunteer or visit a communication support group to practise interaction skills with different clients.

- Do some background reading on the disorders you are most likely to encounter, especially progressive neurological diseases such as Parkinson's disease, MS, MND and dementia.

- Read up on relevant theory, e.g., cognitive neuropsychological models, e.g., Patterson and Shewell, 1987.

- Volunteer in a nursing home to familiarise yourself with the environment and to help develop your skills in talking to a range of clients.

- Make your CE aware of any anxieties you may have, e.g., visiting clients on a hospital ward who are unwell.

- Have a basic awareness of the roles of different members of the MDT. You are likely to work closely within a team so it is important to understand how SLT fits in with other professions.

11 Adults with a traumatic brain injury

Traumatic brain injury (TBI) can be defined as "an alteration in brain function, or evidence of brain pathology, caused by an external force" (Menon, Schwab, Wright, & Maas, 2010). Although prevalence figures vary, severe TBI is estimated to affect 100–150 per 100,000 of the population (Royal Hospital of Neurodisability, 2001). Acceleration–deceleration injuries are one of the most common mechanisms on TBI, during which the person's head is shunted forward at speed and comes to an abrupt halt. The most common cause of these closed head injuries is road traffic accidents (RTAs), which account for between 40–50% of severe TBI (RCSLT, 2006). The injuries suffered can be both focal and diffuse. Diffuse axonal injury can result when neurones are twisted and stretched, and is often associated with dysexecutive symptoms (Constantinidou, Wertheimer, Tsandis, Evan, & Paul, 2012). Focal frontal lobe damage is also common, usually caused by inertial forces propelling the brain forwards against the inside of the skull. Frontal lobe damage frequently results in complex cognitive deficits in addition to speech and language difficulties. These include difficulties with planning and initiation, reduced flexibility of thinking and poor self-awareness and self-regulation (Constantinidou et al., 2012). The range of cognitive-communicative impairments commonly experienced by adults following a TBI can make for a challenging placement, but one which is also highly rewarding. The impacts of reduced insight, low awareness and poor attention on language and communication are complex and varied, and are usually managed by a specialist interdisciplinary team of professionals.

The day-to-day work draws together many of the core academic elements of a speech and language therapy degree: psychology, linguistics, neurology, allowing students to bring their knowledge together and apply it in practice on placement. In this chapter, four students describe the roles that they undertook as a member of an interdisciplinary team in a variety of long-term residential settings. They discuss the complexities of cognitive-communicative deficits and how they both assessed and managed their clients. Finally, several of the students consider the emotional impacts of their placement and how they dealt with the more challenging aspects of their experiences.

Setting

The students were all based in specialist facilities for clients with complex needs following a traumatic brain injury. Chris and Kate spent their placements at residential rehabilitation units, each housing approximately 20 clients. Millie was based in a similar centre that provided specialist services for clients who had acquired cognitive impairments, whereas Jenny spent her placement on a specialist TBI rehabilitation ward within a general hospital.

Despite the students working in similar environments, there was considerable variation in terms of the medical status of their clients, a factor that had a significant impact on the students' daily routines. Jenny worked on a rehabilitation ward with clients who had been transferred there from a regional specialist hospital once they had become medically stable. She was part of a multidisciplinary team who were based on the ward full-time and delivered intensive therapy. Clients who deteriorated or became acutely unwell were transferred back to the specialist hospital rather than being treated on the rehabilitation ward. Consequently, Jenny did not work with clients who were medically unstable, but she did find that the changing medical status of some clients was one of the key challenges of her placement.

> You would make tremendous progress with them, you'd be doing really well and then all of a sudden something would happen. A complex medical event would happen which would not necessarily wipe out [their progress], but [it would] have a tremendous effect on their stability and status. **Jenny**

At the residential rehabilitation unit where Chris spent his placement, the therapies and the majority of the medical care were delivered on-site. Each client had their own private room, which allowed them to personalise their space with their own belongings but also receive the necessary specialist care. One area of the unit was dedicated to clients with the most severe injuries, all of whom had tracheostomies, required ventilation and had 24-hour one-to-one nursing. Another part of the unit was designed to support patients who were less acutely unwell and did not require ventilation. The length of time clients stayed on the rehabilitation unit varied from months to years depending on their status. The unit operated according to a regular daily routine in order to meet the needs of clients who usually had complex and changeable needs.

> There was a handover every day at 9 o'clock. At least one representative of each of the disciplines went along to the nurse's station. The nurse gave us a handover of what happened overnight, how people were doing, if there had been any difficulties, if anyone had been transferred to hospital, which happened if they went into an acute phase. **Chris**

Family and friends were able to visit freely once the nursing staff had helped the clients to be comfortable each morning and each client usually had speech and language therapy, physiotherapy and occupational therapy on a daily basis. Chris explained the importance of residents having 'downtime' throughout each day as a result of the effects of fatigue and that, despite the regular routines, a flexible approach was necessary.

> If the client was going out on a community visit or was going to the hospital, you had to work around that…and you had to have one of the representatives for whatever they were going for…I went out and saw a FEES [flexible endoscopic evaluation of swallowing] being done. **Chris**

Millie also found that she needed to take an organised but flexible approach in terms of her work with clients at the specialist residential unit where she was based for placement.

> We had a breakfast group, so everybody who fed orally went down for their breakfast. All the clients had a timetable, so they would maybe have physio at such a time, then speech therapy. But, say, if we were coming to breakfast group, and there was one member of staff and two clients, maybe those clients needed somebody else to stay on. In that setting your appointment waits. In that situation I thought, "Well, I obviously I need to be here with the other member of staff" and that was how things worked. So you had your appointment times but it was quite flexible, just to meet the needs really, it was just about safety. **Millie**

The students agreed that one of the most important aspects of their placement was developing an understanding of how they fitted into the multidisciplinary team of professionals who worked with the clients.

> It was hugely multidisciplinary. There was social work, a psychologist, OT, physio, SLT. They had a consultant neuro-rehabilitation specialist who came in once a week and then there were all the nursing staff. **Chris**

Although MDT teams operated differently across the various placements, all of the students stressed the importance of close teamwork, which was encouraged by shared open-plan offices. Both Millie and Chris were surprised about the high level of integration between the different professionals but quickly discovered the positive impacts on client care. The students worked as part of an 'interdisciplinary' team (IDT), meaning that all of the professionals had shared client goals and a comprehensive understanding of each other's roles.

> The MDT liaised very, very closely all the time. I thought it might be they got together for a meeting once a week…no, they were constantly talking and chatting about clients. It was so integrated. I had never seen work in any placement as integrated. They liaised very closely in terms of the therapy and the timetabling of the therapy. **Chris**

Multidisciplinary team meetings were a regular part of placement for all of the students although more informal discussions also took place on a daily basis, and Chris found that he needed to adapt his interaction style to suit these different contexts.

> You had the meeting once a week with the consultant, when of course everyone behaves completely differently. We were all sitting around the table in the boardroom and we would all have the files out and we would all be talking very seriously. They were always serious professionals…but usually more relaxed… "So and so is not well at the moment", or "He's having an off day", so there were different levels. I was observing in a way and having to adapt my demeanour according to whichever situation I was in. **Chris**

Millie initially found it challenging to think of herself as part of the team because of her role as a student on placement, but soon found that this was not a barrier to her participation. In fact, taking an active role in meetings was an important aspect of client care.

> They all met once a week to discuss different clients and I was just encouraged to share any relevant information. I was encouraged to be a part of it. I don't know if 'ethical' is the word, but if you knew information about them [the client] and you were in a team meeting, it was your duty to share it. **Millie**

The students felt that working so closely within a team of professionals was an overwhelmingly positive experience, despite initially finding this one of the most daunting aspects of their placement. As they gained in confidence, many of the students found that liaising with other professionals was a two-way process. Not only were they able to gather useful information about their clients, but even as students they were able to make valuable contributions to the work of the other professionals within their team.

> I loved the atmosphere, I loved the care that everybody had for each one of those clients, no matter how difficult they were. They had a huge amount of care and respect for all of the clients. It was a really lovely atmosphere to work in. I liked the interdisciplinary atmosphere, I wouldn't even call it multi [disciplinary], it was interdisciplinary. I loved that. **Chris**

In addition to regular meetings and discussions, the different professionals also developed shared goals and the students often carried out joint sessions with clients. Millie carried out a joint session with the team's occupational therapist who was working on kitchen skills such as cooking.

> I was providing compensatory strategies to aid word finding while the OT worked towards increasing the client's abilities to carry out activities of daily living. I am not trained to help the client with fine motor skills so needed the support of the OT. On the other hand, I was able to provide the OT with strategies to facilitate communication. I think as a student [it was important to think about] what's best for the client and be independent and use your initiative and say, "Right, I'm going to approach the OT and see if she

> would like to do a joint session with me", and not feeling
> timid about doing that. And in the IDT I found they really
> appreciated that and responded well. Those joint sessions
> in the end were really good. **Millie**

Chris worked regularly with therapy assistants who had skills in a range of allied health professions and liaised closely with nursing staff as part of the discharge process.

> There were two clients with locked-in syndrome who were
> both getting ready for discharge... their homes had all been
> adapted. You get a lot of shadowing of nurses who are going
> to be caring at home, because they have got to learn how
> to hoist, how to communicate, how to be tracheostomy
> trained. **Chris**

Caseload

Many of the students found that, although their clients varied hugely in many ways, a significant proportion were young men in their early 20s. Evidence suggests that this is a particularly high-risk demographic for head injury (Rimmel, Jane, & Bond, 1990) and the students found that many of their clients had either been assaulted or involved in a road traffic accident, two of the leading causes of TBI (Powell, 2004). On the residential rehabilitation unit, Kate worked predominantly with young clients who had been physically assaulted.

> I was working with a lad who was 30 who'd been hit across
> the head with an iron bar, an assault. And then there was
> another guy there who was beaten up and thrown out of
> a car. **Kate**

In addition to the more common causes of TBI, several of the students worked with clients whose difficulties had more unusual origins. Jenny worked with a small number of female clients who had experienced ruptured aneurysms during childbirth and Chris worked with one client for whom the aetiology of his symptoms was unknown.

> He was a young man on holiday and experienced significant
> muscle weakness in his legs all of a sudden one day and

> so took himself to hospital. They were querying whether
> it was an insect bite or not. They had never been able to
> establish [the cause] with him. He was able to nod and
> shake his head consistently and he had facial expression
> as well. **Chris**

All of the students gained some experience of working with clients who were nonverbal. Their roles with these clients primarily focused on trialling alternative modes of communication, from low-tech strategies to high-tech devices.

> I only worked with one verbal client. Another client I
> worked with…he was nonverbal and he was having real
> difficulty due to dystonia. He was using 'eye up' for "Yes"
> which seemed to be commonplace. Tongue protrusion for
> "No". They kept happening together and he was having to
> work really, really hard. His jaw was permanently open
> and fixed so there was no possibility of oral movement.
> There was another client who had been a victim of an
> assault and he was making quite a bit of progress but he
> had a tendency to lash out with his arms and limbs by way
> of saying "No".

On the hospital ward, Jenny found that her clients with TBI were being cared for alongside clients with neurodegenerative conditions such as motor neurone disease or multiple sclerosis. She was very aware of the contrast in these two groups of clients; those with TBI were often making some degree of progress compared with clients whose abilities were declining. Millie found that due to the multifocal damage that most of her clients had experienced, each client presented with a highly individual set of difficulties. Jenny and Millie both talked extensively about the complexity and variability of their clients and the challenges that they faced as a result.

> It's not just about the language difficulty. There was a
> real interplay of the social side, the behavioural side, the
> cognitive. Everything interplays within that and adds
> to that communication difficulty. Thinking about the
> cognitive impairment, I think that is massive. Don't just
> have an aphasia language hat on…realise how everything
> interlinks. I think that is so important. **Millie**

Although lectures and background reading had prepared the students for placement to some extent, it was still a challenge to plan for all of the variables that often impacted on a session with a client following a head injury.

> You had to really have several hats on when you were with the client, so you've got your speech and language therapy hat on…but you also had to take into account cognition. You had to take into account that fatigue levels influence [performance]. You had to be sensitive to distractions. So not to attribute responses solely to speech and language difficulties. **Jenny**

The students found that taking a very flexible approach to their interaction and therapy helped them to build rapport with their clients and enable the most positive outcomes. They found that clients varied enormously from one another in terms of their level of functioning, but also that the performance of individual clients often varied within the same day as a result of factors such as fatigue, motivation and cognition. Jenny worked with one client who displayed enormous variation depending on who he was interacting with, something which presented a significant challenge for the speech and language therapy team and which emphasises the importance of observing and interacting with clients in a range of different contexts in order to build an accurate profile of their abilities.

> We were assessing a man who [had] very, very low awareness and [his] prognosis was not terrific. We could assess that he was tracking and possibly moving to sound…he had no expressive language, no functional swallow. But his family were presenting a different picture and saying that he was speaking and turning and saying "Mum". That's where you have to pick it apart. The family desperately want to see progress so "Mum" is very easy to misinterpret [when it] is just an involuntary vocalisation. So we did a couple of observations and there was nothing, no consistency for us and then the SLT deliberately went in when the family were there, as the family entered, just to see, and he turned and he said, "Mum". **Jenny**

The complex and unpredictable nature of this client group presented a challenge for the students, but this aspect of placement was also one of the most enjoyable. The students faced new challenges every day and relished the problem-solving aspect of working with their clients.

> It's an incredibly complex, multifaceted puzzle and you need to keep in sight that, as much as you'd like to spend the rest of your life unpicking that person's puzzle, they need to be at a level of functionality and that's what we're aiming for. So always keep your goals in sight so you don't get distracted by..."That's really interesting, why are you doing that?" **Jenny**

Frontal lobe damage was one of the most common injuries suffered by clients on the students' caseloads. These injuries commonly result in changes to communication, behaviour regulation and a range of executive functions, all of which interplay to create a multifaceted set of symptoms. The students all found it challenging to work with clients who presented with cognitive-communicative deficits. The inherent difficulties involved in teasing apart a client's underlying impairments can sometimes be addressed by multidisciplinary teamwork. Joint sessions or sharing information in team meetings often revealed information that drastically altered the types of input and intervention being offered to the client. In one such case, Jenny carried out a joint session with a social worker, which revealed that their client had a far more significant cognitive impairment than she had previously thought.

> The social worker pushed cognitive questions that we hadn't thought to investigate because previous presentation had indicated that her cognitive skills were fine. The social worker said, "Do you know where you are?" She [the client] replied in the best way she could, in fact her body language was very much, "I know where I am" and if I were the social worker, I would have left it. The social worker asked, "Are you in a school, a hospital or home?" And I thought she was going to automatically say "hospital", but she paused and paused a lot longer and my stomach hit the ground and she said, "I don't know", so we then started to do further cognitive investigation. **Jenny**

One of the most common cognitive deficits that clients presented with was a lack of insight into their own abilities and limitations. The effects of this were highly dependent on the individual and ranged enormously in terms of magnitude. For example, Jenny described one client who had highly unrealistic expectations of his own abilities due to a lack of insight.

> He said, "I can go home, I can walk the dog, no problem." This is somebody that can't get out of his wheelchair. **Jenny**

The impacts of poor insight and awareness were an everyday challenge and influenced both therapy and the emotional presentation of clients. Chris found that a lack of insight often led to behaviours that were difficult for the MDT to manage and raised a number of ethical questions.

> One challenging client insisted that she didn't need ventilating and became hypoxic. She was adamant that she knew what was wrong with her and everybody else was wrong if they told her otherwise and she was very much in control of when she went on the vent [ventilator] and when she needed the vent. That comes under capacity. Does the client actually have capacity and does that capacity vary depending on how well or not they are? **Chris**

Millie found that reduced self-awareness and insight meant that some clients did not experience the levels of frustration or emotions that she had expected because they lacked understanding about their situation. Those clients who were unaware of their communication difficulties were often much less motivated to engage with therapy. Although a lack of insight was a common feature of many clients, this was not the case for everybody. Chris, Jenny and Millie all worked regularly with at least one client who had locked-in syndrome following brainstem injury. People with locked-in syndrome are conscious, but present with quadriplegia, anarthria, dysphagia and lack of facial expression (Garrard et al., 2002). In addition, executive function, memory and attention span are often impaired. Communication is usually achieved by vertical eye movement, though vision can be impaired, and clients with locked-in syndrome have an awareness of their difficulties which creates a unique set of challenges in terms of speech and language therapy.

> They'll have insight into the fact that they're not doing as well as they would like, and are frustrated by that and they

have unrealistic expectations [about] what can be achieved in therapy and what they can actually do. **Jenny**

Millie found that she was often able to address some of the unpredictable behaviours by adjusting her approach to interacting with her clients.

> Often the clients can be very impulsive. So maybe if something wasn't done right, when they wanted it, there'd be a bit of behavioural [change]. But I think often what worked for me as a student was just approaching it right… coming down to their level and understanding what it is that was causing the behaviour and working on that. Treating the individual as an equal partner…talking it through with them and seeing maybe what they think is best. I think when I did that, they responded really well, so that really helped. **Millie**

One of the most common complications following TBI is post-traumatic amnesia, which can persist for days or months following the injury and have a significant impact on the delivery of therapy. Around 70% of people develop anterograde amnesia following TBI (Tate et al., 2006), which affects the ability to learn and recall new information and can make therapy particularly challenging for both clients and the team of professionals. Several of the students found it challenging to build a relationship with clients and to design effective therapy for their clients with amnesia, often finding that a functional approach and regular sessions were the most effective means of delivery for these clients.

> He [the client] didn't remember me from one day to the next and he found it very difficult to learn new tasks cognitively. **Chris**

Client assessment

The majority of client assessment was carried out informally, either using informal screening tests or behavioural observation. There is a wealth of evidence to support this approach, which further suggests that as post-traumatic amnesia reduces, more formal assessments can be introduced (Constantinidou et al., 2012). Millie found that informal assessment was a vital method of gauging how clients behaved and communicated in a functional way during the acute stages post-TBI.

> It was really, really important to do informal assessment. Difficulties in 'real world' situations can be disguised by formal assessments which usually don't investigate language past the sentence level. Individualised informal assessments and observations of clients in functional and social settings is essential. **Millie**

Chris also found that formal assessments were not suitable for his clients with low levels of awareness and that much of the acute assessment consisted of regular observations to monitor any small signs of progress. He also discovered that it was important to understand the key assessments used by other professionals in the MDT because the results could influence his work with clients. The Wessex Head Injury Matrix (Shiel, Wilson, McLellan, Watson, & Horn, 2000) was a common assessment used by psychologists to measure cognitive function following head injury and Chris found that these results informed his approach to both interaction and intervention with clients.

Both Chris and Jenny worked with clients who had dysphagia and were involved to varying extents with the assessment of their clients' swallow. Chris tended to observe his CE carrying out informal bedside dysphagia screens, whereas Jenny was able to play a more active role in feeling and listening to the swallow using a stethoscope and gained insight into the complexities involved in screening for dysphagia.

> [You need to] be aware that there is a person in front of you who is about to [undergo] an unpleasant procedure, so reassure them, try to still connect with them. Stop trying to see only the sounds they are making, but the individual they are. Try to juggle all of that, because you are spending so much time going, "Am I holding the cup right…can I hear it properly?" that you forget that this person is desperate to eat, is trying to please you so that they can eat and is about to aspirate. So it's all very complex. **Jenny**

The students all found that assessing clients offered them a fascinating insight into the complexity and unique nature of the effects of TBI, though they stressed the importance of having sound rationale for the types of assessment that they chose to conduct.

> You can just keep delving, keep assessing, keep unpicking and you have to be careful about whether the unpicking is

informing functional therapy and your goals or whether it's just satisfying your own curiosity or your own exploration as to why it might be happening, so always keep your goals in sight. **Jenny**

Intervention

The students used a range of intervention approaches with their clients. Some clients received impairment-based therapy, whereas others benefitted from a more functional approach, often using AAC methods. Most of the therapy techniques were akin to those used with any client who has an acquired communication impairment; however, the students found that clients with TBI often presented them with a unique set of challenges. Rapidly changing medical status, post-traumatic amnesia and the emotional impacts on both the client and their families all contributed to the complexity of designing and implementing effective therapy programmes.

Although all of the students were involved to some degree with clients who had dysphagia, most of their day-to-day work focused on addressing their clients' language impairments. Kate used the cognitive neuropsychological model (Patterson & Shewell, 1987) as a basis for designing therapy and, despite her initial reservations, she felt that it provided a useful basis for moving through a hierarchy of tasks with her clients.

I know the cognitive neuropsychological model like the back of my hand now. I was doing the auditory phonological analysis down to semantics. So I was doing minimal pairs, spoken word-picture matching, written word-picture matching. Because he had no output, we didn't go any further, we just got as far as semantics, and obviously lexical decisions as well. I actually really liked it. It makes sense. It's logical and it also helps you plan your therapy and it did give me a really clear overview of what I want to do. **Kate**

Millie and Chris both worked regularly with clients who presented with anomia (word-finding difficulties). Whilst Millie's therapy primarily focused on word-finding strategies at a single-word level, Chris worked at a sentence level with a client who had just been admitted onto the rehabilitation unit.

> She was challenging, she was new in whilst I was there and they were trying to stabilise her. She was high level… complaining of word-finding difficulties, she had no swallow, she [had a tracheostomy], she was ventilated, but she was mobile. We were looking at word-finding difficulties using Stackhouse and Wells [Stackhouse & Wells, 1997] which didn't work. She was adamant she had word-finding problems so we used Garrett's model[32] at the message and functional levels of sentence production rather than a single word level. **Chris**

Alongside this more traditional impairment-based approach, all of the students worked towards functional goals with some of their clients. This took many forms and was highly specific to individual clients. Jenny encouraged her clients to use gesture, drawing and writing to support their expressive language. Millie found that she needed to introduce specific strategies for her client with memory difficulties and encouraged generalisation of these strategies by taking her client outside of the residential unit.

> We needed to make it a lot more functional, rather than just sitting showing pictures, and [explaining] the strategy. So what I liked to do at the start of every session was a recap of the materials. Especially for somebody who maybe isn't going to remember what you're doing and can use the strategies but doesn't remember how to use them. Each time, I was lessening my prompting and seeing if the client did use a bit more of their initiative. So your sessions became quite long. You weren't having your thirty minutes, you were going to the supermarket and seeing if they could remember what was on their list and [using] the strategies. **Millie**

Kate also accompanied her clients on trips out of the rehabilitation unit, visiting a local pet shop with a client who was due to be discharged and wanted an aquarium at home. She encouraged him to use the communication strategies that they had been working on to speak to local shopkeepers and buy the necessary equipment.

---

32   Garrett, M.F. (1988). Processes in language production. In F.I. Newmeyer (Ed.), *Linguistics: The Cambridge survey: III. Language: Psychological and biological aspects.* Cambridge: Cambridge University Press.

In addition to working with verbal clients, all of the students worked with some nonverbal clients during their placement. In many cases, their work involved iintroducing AAC devices and helping their client to build skills and confidence in using these new modes of communication. Kate worked with several clients who had locked-in syndrome, using both low- and high-tech AAC devices.

> Two locked-in syndrome clients used auditory alphabet. One on a frequency level and the other just going through "abcd". They had also just got an [eye-tracking device] on trial for four weeks to try with one of the locked-in clients because his eye gaze was good. I also saw him in an OT session using a chin switch to change channel on his TV. **Kate**

Millie also worked with clients to introduce AAC. Part of her role was to train the client's family members to understand the devices and optimise their own communication skills. Many of the students had regular contact with the family and friends of their clients, either at case conferences or during visiting hours. Jenny found that dealing with the emotions of both her clients and their family was one of the most challenging aspects of her placement and that there was a significant impact of the emotional status of clients on their progress in therapy.

> That's the tricky thing with this placement, the emotional impact it can have in the respect that these people are grieving, both their family and themselves, and you need to be aware of that grief and how it is impacting on the therapy and that you don't exacerbate it. You keep them motivated. I did it through balancing tasks I knew he would do well in, with tasks I knew he would struggle with. A relatively easy task which was still targeting elements I wanted to do and reactivating memories and language, but giving him the confidence to then do the next task that he really really struggled with. Then I would end with a task that I knew he would sail through, so that he came out really positive from that therapy session. **Jenny**

The changing medical status of some clients had a significant impact on their ability to engage with therapy and the degree of recovery of their communication skills. For some clients, they became gradually more medically stable, whereas others experienced setbacks which influenced their language recovery. Kate assessed one client on her last day of placement and described the sudden change in his performance.

> He hadn't really been having any speech and language therapy because he was so low level. The consultant had taken him off one of his medications or given him another medication…so it was the third day of this and he was far more alert and awake so we went in to try to assess him, because we hadn't even been able to do that. We got consistent looking up at the ceiling for "Yes" and orientating to the door. We just came out afterwards and were jumping up and down. It was so lovely. **Kate**

In contrast, Jenny worked with a client who experienced post-traumatic seizures, which led to setbacks in her communication skills and emotional status.

> The patient's health is a very important factor in therapy. Her comprehension appeared to be relatively intact and we thought her cognition was of an adequate level as well. She was making very good progress. Unfortunately, she had a seizure…and I went into the session unaware of this, which emphasises the need for multidisciplinary working and always keeping up-to-date with the [medical] notes. I'd come in the next day, didn't read the notes. A huge mistake because it said she'd had a seizure and I could have really done with knowing that because she went from doing really well to horrendous, hardly any expressive language. I had to absolutely think on my feet and start again and also give her a little bit of a counselling session because she was very insecure about the deterioration and so the planned session got abandoned so we did something else. **Jenny**

Discussing progress in therapy with a client was a demanding aspect of working with clients who had experienced TBI. The students found that many of their clients were frustrated, upset or angry about what had happened to them and that this could have an impact on their progress in therapy. Jenny talked to her clients about working towards an 'optimum level' and found that this terminology fostered a positive environment without giving her clients unrealistic expectations in terms of their likely recovery. She worked closely with one client who was finding it very difficult to come to terms with his situation and the sudden enormous changes in his life.

> He was getting particularly distressed in my session and I was trying to reassure without generating false expectations. Attempting to encourage and emphasise his progress, whilst reiterating the reality of that progress. He said he was desperate to go home and he wasn't ready to go home. You've got to think of the grieving process, the anger, the self-recrimination, the need to blame others. You know what, they need to feel empowered, because they are currently powerless to an extent. So one way to mediate that is to involve them in therapy, and it's very important to constantly update them, to make them aware of what's going on. But to be aware of their emotional vulnerability as well. So, always have that at the back of your mind. Sometimes their outbursts need to happen and they're not necessarily directed at you, they're just an expression of their emotion. You need to help them express that emotion so it's being aware that none of it's personal. **Jenny**

Over the course of a block placement, many of the students witnessed significant degrees of recovery in terms of their clients' overall functioning and found this a hugely rewarding aspect of their placements. Some clients made very small steps towards recovery, whereas others showed a substantial improvement in their communication skills. Millie found that her client's cognitive impairments had a huge impact on their progress, but that once she had adjusted to these factors, the outcomes were very encouraging.

> Due to the cognitive difficulties, attention and lack of initiative...you're really doing a lot of the same things in every session, so you'd find that the progress was quite slow, but that even the smallest step was a great improvement. So you're not looking for great improvements, even small things, you're like, "Oh brilliant." It was a real encouragement. **Millie**

Chris worked with a client who was admitted to the rehabilitation unit shortly after he had started placement. Due to the nature of block placements, he was able to work regularly with the gentleman and observe him make significant improvements in function.

> When he came in, he was completely globally aphasic, PEG-fed, couldn't move, couldn't talk, couldn't do anything. When we'd finished working with him after eight weeks… his understanding was better, it wasn't within normal limits, but his understanding was better. His expressive language was still very impaired, but he could communicate, he could walk, he could eat proper food. It was amazing his recovery, absolutely amazing. That was a very rewarding part of the placement. **Chris**

Emotional impacts

All of the students were prepared for a placement that would be emotionally challenging due to the nature of their clients' injuries and circumstances. Some found this aspect more difficult to deal with than others, but all described the high levels of support that they received, not only from their clinical educators but also from the wider MDT. Jenny described a particularly demanding session with one client and how she liaised with her team to provide him with the best support possible.

> This multidisciplinary team were very supportive and I did come out [of a therapy session] and say this client had really expressed a wish to not be here any more. It was hard, because I'd formed a strong relationship with him. Even though that was where his mood was headed, the deterioration of his mood was quite extreme over the weeks. He could talk to me more about it, I think, because it was a communicative session and because I always ended the session with "How are you doing?" I did walk away feeling that my counselling skills were inadequate…I went straight away and found the counsellor. **Jenny**

The students all felt very apprehensive about their placements initially, but were surprised at how quickly they gained confidence and skills. Working with clients who could be acutely unwell remained a challenge, but this did become a little easier as the students grew accustomed the rehabilitation environment over the course of their placements.

> It was a steep learning curve, it was really, really steep... adapting to the client group, working really, really hard to have a good rapport and not appear patronising whilst learning on your feet. Interpersonal skills were a real challenge for me, you know, not to appear upset or disturbed. It's a challenge. **Chris**

Building rapport with their clients was one of the most rewarding aspects of placement for the students, despite this being an initial concern given the complexities of the client group. Most of the clients were long-term residents in the rehabilitation setting and the students often saw their clients for therapy twice per day, enabling them to build up strong relationships. Chris reflected on the contrast between the emotional impact on him compared with the reactions of his client's family.

> I didn't know them in a pre-morbid state...I wasn't emotionally attached to that person but I very quickly became emotionally attached to the post-morbid person. **Chris**

Millie learned that it was vital not to make assumptions about her client's emotional wellbeing and state of mind. She worked regularly with a client with locked-in syndrome, and Millie soon found that her client had a very positive state of mind, despite initial assumptions that her client was likely to be feeling unhappy. Millie also talked about treading a fine line between empathy and maintaining her professional role. She found that she often discussed her feelings with her MDT and peers, because it was not appropriate to express her emotions in front of her clients and their families.

> I thought it was going to be hard emotionally and that was actually quite tough... really getting the balance between being a human and having a heart, but then realising I was a professional there to help, not to reduce the effectiveness of my therapy because of getting overly emotional. I think you really just value people when they're in their situations, so I think it is emotional but if you take the right approach you can definitely really enjoy it. **Millie**

Summary

The students all agreed that their placements working with clients following head injury were among the most rewarding, challenging and varied that they had experienced during their degree course. Despite initial concerns about how they would build relationships with clients and manage the possible emotions involved in working with people who are unwell, they all gave an overwhelmingly positive account of their time on placement.

> I loved the type of therapies that were done. I loved the fact we could get out and about, I loved the different levels, I loved the different requirements of each client. I loved the fact that we could go out into the community and do visits, we could go to the hospital and do a videofluoroscopy. **Kate**

Top tips from students

- Prepare by reading your lecture notes and carry out your own further reading about TBI. Continue reading throughout your placement so that you can integrate the theory into your management of clients.

- Remember that cognitive difficulties often have a significant impact on therapy outcomes. A client may perform well in the session, but may not demonstrate retention from one session to the next, so progress may be slow. Often even very small steps are considered great improvements.

- Generalisation of skills to outside of the therapy sessions is often poor, so therapy tasks of a very functional nature are often the most useful.

- The interdisciplinary team is so important. Make sure that you liaise closely with other disciplines and work towards shared goals. Share your own specialist knowledge whilst taking on information from the other specialists.

- Try not to think with your 'aphasia hat' on! Although there may be similar language impairments, they are usually more intertwined with cognitive, behavioural and social changes in TBI.

- It is essential to incorporate informal assessments and observation into the assessment process, and to observe your clients interacting in a range of settings. Often individuals with TBI will demonstrate marked difficulties with functional communication and commonly display significant communication impairments in social settings.

Top tips from clinical educators

- Read up on cognitive-communicative disorders and be aware of how these will affect all aspects of the patient's life.

- Have a good knowledge of the roles of occupational therapists and psychologists, particularly in relation to cognitive assessment and activities of daily living.

- Learn about your client from their friends and family. Try to tailor your therapy to their interests to make it more relevant and motivating. Be creative!

- Don't feel under pressure to 'perform' in therapy sessions, especially with low awareness clients. You can often learn more from just observing them during their morning routine or in a physiotherapy session and this counts as part of your informal assessment.

- Work closely with other therapists, support each other. For example, work with the OT for positioning for feeding, or the music therapist for breathing or voice work. Make the most of joint sessions to learn from each other.

- Prepare yourself for working with families. It won't be easy, but they need support and information. Keep them updated on your input and get them involved where possible.

- Be prepared to think flexibly. Many patients with severe cognitive-communicative impairment do not suit a test-therapy-retest model. Be aware that the SLT role can be in disability management rather than direct therapy, e.g., working with families to create life books.

12 Voice

Clients with voice disorders may either present with aphonia, an inability to produce any voice, or dysphonia, an impairment to phonation. Dysphonia is often characterised by a change to voice quality, for example, a client may present with a creaky or hoarse voice. Changes to pitch, volume and resonance may also be apparent. Voice disorders range greatly in their severity and the psychosocial impacts are equally varied depending on the client's occupation, social environment and emotional status. Incidence and prevalence figures vary enormously, with some research suggesting that the incidence in the UK is as high as 121 per 100,000 (Mathieson, 2001). Prevalence figures are consistently highest among professional voice users, for example teachers, call centre workers, barristers or performers. Many studies have reported evidence to suggest that teachers make up a significant proportion of a voice clinic caseload, with incidence figures estimated to be as high as 38% amongst this population (Smith, Lemke, Taylor, Kirchner, & Hoffman, 1998). There has been much debate in the literature about the classification of voice disorders, leading to many systems that vary internationally. The most widely-used system of classification in the UK is a multifactorial model (Enderby et al., 2009a), which recognises the interactions between four distinct aetiologies: inflammation, structural, muscle tension and neuromuscular. Voice disorders may result from any one or a combination of these aetiologies.

Most students will encounter clients with a voice disorder during their time on clinical placements. Many join a multidisciplinary team based in a specialist clinic and spend their placement working solely with clients who present with dysphonia or aphonia. Some students will also gain experience of working with clients with dysphonia as part of a general caseload of adults who have acquired neurological impairments or, more rarely, as part of a paediatric caseload. This chapter focuses on the experience of five students, all of whom had an adult caseload, but in a variety of settings.

In this chapter, the students consider their role as a speech and language therapy student within a specialist multidisciplinary team. They recall their experiences of taking client case histories and conducting subsequent assessments. The students also reflect on the wide range of clients they worked with on their placements, and the most common intervention approaches that they used to address dysphonia.

Setting

The students all spent at least some of their placement in a specialist voice outpatient clinic within a hospital. Two students also made home visits to see clients in addition to their regular clinics. Although primarily hospital-based, the diversity of student experiences clearly demonstrates the range of ways in which voice services are run across the UK. Eliza spent her placement in a clinic run as a collaborative venture by both SLTs and specialist ear, nose and throat doctors (also known as otolaryngologists). Joint clinics are becoming increasingly common the UK. Otolaryngologists and SLTs work collaboratively using their own areas of expertise and specific skills to assess, diagnose and treat the voice problem (Enderby et al., 2009a). Sarah worked solely with a team of SLTs at a hospital, receiving almost all client referrals from the ear, nose and throat department (ENT) but without any direct contact or meetings with ENT. The other students worked primarily with SLTs, but attended occasional joint ENT clinics. Both Eliza and Georgina reflected positively on their experiences of working with and learning from other professionals. They gained a much deeper understanding of the SLT role in this environment and how their work linked with the roles of other professionals in the MDT. Both found that the hospital environment suited their working styles and began to feel like part of the team as their placements progressed.

> I loved it [the outpatient clinical setting]. I liked the variation. I liked the way everything was quick. Everyone knew what they were doing, everyone worked well as a team. **Georgina**

Some of the other students found that their experiences were quite repetitive and lacked the variation described by Georgina. Despite this apparent criticism, they actually felt that this was a positive aspect of their placement because they could track their own personal development and gained personal satisfaction with the progress that they were making in terms of their clinical skills. They also felt that because of the repetitive nature of some aspects, for example writing case notes, their CE developed higher expectations in line with the experience and practice that they were gaining.

There was great variety in terms of how frequently clients attended appointments at the voice clinics. Some clients attended just for initial assessment and were then referred to another professional, such as a psychologist. All of the students gained some experience of seeing clients through from initial assessment to discharge. Many felt that this was a particularly rewarding and interesting aspect to their experience and something that they had gained little experience of on previous placements. Block placements allowed the students to see a client for their initial assessment, followed by weekly therapy sessions for 4–6 weeks, leading to discharge from the service. Due to the high proportion of employed professional voice users on the caseload, Georgina discovered that some clients attended appointments outside of normal working hours so that they were not required to take time off work.

The three students who worked in a joint ENT clinic were all extremely positive about their experiences, despite initially finding it a daunting prospect. They were surprised to find that the specialist SLTs often conducted the nasendoscopies themselves, which the students were able to observe. Prior to the procedure, Eliza handed out questionnaires to clients to gain their perception of their voice. She then worked alongside her CE to take a case history and carry out the GRBAS rating scale (Hirano, 1981) to provide a baseline measure of vocal quality. Following a local anaesthetic, the SLT conducted the nasendoscopy with Eliza observing the procedure.

> We actually did endoscopies and we saw quite a lot of patients with cancer and some patients that had nodules and polyps. And we actually got to see those, I didn't expect that at all, that was amazing. You'd look at the vocal cords, and you'd obviously be able to tell if there was any inflammation or anything, and then the speech therapists would talk about it and then go to the ENT consultant. He would come in and then would say if he thought [the client should have] speech therapy or surgery. Sometimes I suppose it was hard, because sometimes mucus you thought could be a nodule or a polyp. So sometimes they had to cough a few times. If it was a suspected polyp, then straight away [they would have] surgery just in case it was cancer. **Eliza**

Georgina also liaised closely with other professionals at a joint endoscopy clinic. She primarily worked alongside otolaryngologists and speech and language therapy assistants and found that the roles of the different professionals on the MDT were very clearly defined.

There was a specialist doctor that had to confirm the SLT's findings and then they'd sign it off. We worked very closely with the speech therapy assistant who would set up all the equipment. And, obviously I guess, if there was a lot of psychological trauma associated with the voice, then they might refer them to a psychologist. **Georgina**

All of the students involved in MDT work felt that they learned a great deal from this collaborative style of working. During the early stages of their placements, many of the students were particularly anxious about working so closely with professionals from other disciplines and found this to be quite an intimidating experience. However, they adjusted quickly as they gained knowledge, skills and confidence. Those students who did not work directly with other professionals found that they still liaised regularly with the ENT department, but that this was usually via telephone conversations as opposed to regular meetings. They also received medical reports such as endoscopy results from ENT, and were involved in assisting their CE to write reports and referrals to other departments within the hospital.

Caseload

Perhaps one of the most unique aspects of a voice placement is the wide range in the age of clients on the caseload. Although research suggests that voice disorders most commonly occur between the ages of 40 and 59 years (Roy, Stemple, Merrill, & Thomas, 2005), a caseload commonly spans from children through to an elderly population. All of the students interviewed worked solely with adults, with the youngest aged 16 and the eldest aged 91. Not only did their clients encompass a range of ages but they also presented with a huge range of diagnoses, leading to an extremely varied caseload for many of the students. Voice disorders can result from changes to the larynx, vocal tract, respiratory or neurological systems. The causes are equally diverse, including physical or psychological trauma, infection, cancer, neurological disease and vocal abuse. The students found that the range of aetiologies led to a varied and interesting caseload.

The students all gained some experience working with clients who had voice disorders of a psychogenic origin. Voice is used to express emotions and, consequently, feelings of anxiety, stress or depression can lead to transient changes to the voice, for example a higher pitch or decrease in volume. Vocal changes such as these can persist beyond the emotional state and lead to long-term psychogenic aphonia or dysphonia. Whilst some students commented on the fact that the placement was exactly what they had expected from a voice caseload, Ann found that the impacts of dysphonia varied according to the individual.

> I don't think it's predictable at all because everyone's got different reasons why they come to you and reasons for why it's happened, so you're still going to be targeting different things. **Ann**

The students reported that the most common types of voice disorder that they observed on placement were presbyphonia, vocal changes related to Parkinson's disease, psychogenic dysphonia, hoarse voice caused by reflux, and muscle tension dysphonia, which often led to secondary organic changes. Most of the students worked with elderly clients who presented with age-related voice changes known as presbyphonia. These changes are caused by a decrease in muscle tone in the laryngeal and respiratory muscles as a result of normal ageing and can affect pitch, volume and voice quality. Like all voice disorders, the range and severity of the impacts on a person's life can vary enormously depending on the individual. Some elderly clients reported that they were no longer able to sing at church as a result of the changes in their voice, whereas for others, presbyphonia had more general impacts on their social interactions.

> In the case of the little old lady, she'd be chatting to her friends like she used to be able to but you know, muscles deteriorates a bit with age and her breath support wasn't quite as good as it used to be. **Rob**

Several students also worked frequently with clients who had Parkinson's disease. The most common changes to the voice in Parkinson's disease are low volume and a monotonous quality, both of which are often targets for speech and language therapy. However, it is also important to view every client holistically and not just focus on the medical condition. Sarah described a particularly complex case of a client with early-onset Parkinson's disease.

> She was really quite fragile and there was more going on
> than could be explained by her Parkinson's and her [early]
> stage of Parkinson's. And she was obviously quite upset
> and distressed. **Sarah**

This case highlights something discussed by several students: that often
there is a complex interaction of factors in a client's life which can lead to or
exacerbate a voice disorder. Many were surprised about how frequently there
was a psychogenic element to a client's dysphonia. All found that working
with clients who presented with psychogenic dysphonia was one of the most
challenging elements to their placement, but also one of the most interesting
because they were able to draw on their knowledge of psychology.

> I find that link fascinating between psychology and how
> that can affect your physiology. That absolutely fascinates
> me, it always has. **Sarah**

All had some opportunity to work directly with clients presenting with
psychogenic dysphonia; however, in some cases, they observed sessions
led by their CE and discussed these more complex clients after the session.
Stress was one of the most frequent factors in the case history of this client
group. Many studies have demonstrated the links between stress and muscle
tension, which frequently leads to muscle tension dysphonia (Deary, Wilson,
Carding, & Mackenzie, 2003; Demmink-Geertman & Dejonckere, 2002).
Though stress can be a causal factor, the voice disorder itself then often
leads to further stress because of its impacts on a person's work and social
life. Many of the students discovered that sessions with these clients could
be emotionally demanding, particularly if their clients became upset, which
happened relatively frequently.

> I was doing humming work with her with the letter 'm'
> and one of the words was 'mother' and she broke down in
> the session. It was a bit of a breakthrough, but at the same
> time it was very shocking. I asked her if she was OK and
> got her a glass of water and an opportunity to chat and
> the session was cancelled. She did open up a tiny bit. It
> turns out that her mother had died several years ago and
> she hadn't really resolved that. It was kind of suppressed…
> obviously, when that lady felt so strongly that she cried in
> the session, that was quite emotional. There was quite often

a psychological cause and when you hear about that, some were more severe than others, but obviously that might impact on you. **Georgina**

Many of the students found that reflux was a very common condition amongst the clinical population and some of the clinics had developed a standard questionnaire to help diagnose reflux. The students regularly carried out this questionnaire with their clients and found that the most common symptoms were a hoarse or rough voice, frequent throat clearing, a dry throat and frequent episodes of wakefulness throughout the night.

> Reflux was quite common. Some people were coming in already with a diagnosis and taking medication…there was no proven link that the condition was causing voice problems but that was the assumption. **Sarah**

All of the students saw professional voice users frequently during their placements. Most were teachers, call centre workers, singers or sports coaches. A diagnosis of muscle tension dysphonia was the most common among this client group, often leading to secondary organic changes such as vocal fold nodules, polyps or haemorrhages. Depending on how the clinic was run, clients had already been seen and diagnosed by ENT, or these changes were detected during a joint ENT and SLT clinic. Georgina discovered that teachers were often unable to get time off to attend blocks of therapy during working hours and so frequently missed their sessions. The students commonly worked with clients who presented with a range of risk factors for dysphonia, such as jobs, hobbies and lifestyles that led to high vocal demand.

> She was a music teacher who never had any breaks, so she was singing and she was a teacher. Then I found out she had 2-year-old twins, then she also coached football in the week. So that was like a typical case. **Eliza**

Many of the clients had been for voice therapy previously and were re-referred for a number of reasons, most commonly that they had forgotten the techniques they had previously used and their dysphonia had returned, or there had been changes in their lifestyle that had exacerbated their voice disorders.

> I think it was due to stress…, or if it was teachers, perhaps they were teaching quite a lot. Or singers, they were having a few more gigs. **Georgina**

The students also worked with clients who presented with particularly complex difficulties or sets of circumstances. They found that taking a detailed case history from clients was crucial in terms of gaining all of the relevant background information so that an accurate diagnosis and appropriate advice could be provided.

> I mean they're all very complex but I think that the main thing that you don't realise until you start doing it a bit is that there's a large number of factors that can contribute [to a voice disorder]. **Rob**

Taking a case history

The students all talked extensively about taking client case histories and reported that this was one of their major roles throughout placement. The case history was taken in the initial session and usually took around one hour, though some could run over a number of sessions if clients had a complex background or if they found it difficult to speak for long periods due to their voice disorder. All of the students used a standard form provided by their CE, but found that they needed to make rapid on-line decisions about which questions were appropriate for individual clients.

> You would just play it by ear, whether you ask every question or not. Just like any case history isn't it, sometimes you think no, that's just not relevant now and you know you're going to see them again and those issues can still be explored later on. **Sarah**

Like many of the students, Rob found that some case histories could take a long time and that it was important not to rush clients through this process. He conducted a particularly challenging case history with a client who had aphonia and consequently needed to write down most of their responses to the questions.

> It took longer than any other case history I'd ever done. Just because there was a lot of stuff to find out really, you needed to get background on how they use their voice at work, at home, stressors and emotional factors, any medical

problems, because they might have been overlooked as well. So it can take quite a long time. **Rob**

Taking a detailed and personal case history from a new client was one of the most difficult aspects of placements in a voice clinic. Some of the students felt uncomfortable about asking personal questions and felt pressure to build up a rapport very quickly with new clients. They found that the clients' reactions to case history questions varied enormously; some clients were surprised at the types of questions they were asked and could be reticent about discussing personal issues.

> I did sometimes get the look of, "Why are you asking me this", but I found that if I explained why it was that I was asking certain things, I got better responses from them. **Ann**

The students agreed that being able to explain and justify their reasons for asking particular questions was critical in terms of putting their client at ease. Many developed their own introductions to a case history session, which they used to help their clients to feel more comfortable.

> You introduce it as, "We're going to ask you some questions, some of them might seem quite personal but, hopefully, when we go through how your voice works, you'll get a bit more of an understanding as to why I'm asking them." **Sarah**

Despite the challenges involved, most of the students enjoyed the process of getting to know their client during the initial session and found that taking an in-depth case history really helped them to get to know their clients and to build strong rapport. The students were then able to use the detailed information to formulate hypotheses about causal factors and a diagnosis that they could then discuss with their clinical educator. Rather than finding this process repetitive, the students felt that the frequency with which they took case histories really helped them to build their clinical skills and gain a range of experience of the different types of voice disorders.

> It was different answers that people were giving, so then you were becoming better at making your diagnosis, or predicting what you were going to see. **Eliza**

Taking a case history from clients with a suspected psychogenic voice disorder was a particularly anxiety-provoking experience, especially during the early stage of the students' placements when they had little experience of working with these complex clients. One of the most challenging aspects was achieving the difficult balance between obtaining key information and maintaining a sensitive approach towards their client. Many practised taking case histories with their friends and family before their placement so that they could find the best way to word questions and ask them in a sensitive manner. Despite this, some students found that it could take a number of weeks for their clients to feel sufficiently comfortable to share personal information.

> I did feel like I needed to take some time [to] develop the relationship. If you establish a good rapport to start then anything that's relevant will come out. And it's true that two or three weeks in, I was still learning things about my client. **Sarah**

Some clients were open and willing to answer all of the case history questions, offering lots of detail without much prompting from the student. Others were more reluctant to discuss their past in detail, but the students agreed that this was something they adjusted to over the period of their placement and, as they gained experience, they became much more adept at judging the emotional status of their clients.

> It can be sort of spotting just when actually they don't have much to tell you, compared to they do have stuff to tell you, but they just don't want to go into it. And also a fine line between…do you just leave it until later, or kind of delve into it a bit more, push. Although if you ask slightly more specific questions I think people do come up with better, more specific answers. **Rob**

Assessment

The students agreed that a case history was the most fundamental aspect of gauging a client's difficulties and sometimes this alone formed the basis for diagnosis and intervention. Those who did carry out quantitative assessment in addition to the case history all followed a set protocol of standard outcome measures which was carried out with each client. Most students reported that measuring maximum phonation length of /a:/, pitch scales and volume range were the most common approaches to initial assessment following the case history and allowed them to record a baseline prior to therapy. Some initially felt uncomfortable modelling and recording these assessments, but became used to the assessments as they gained experience.

> It took a bit to get into at first, but then it was absolutely fine. Just because if people think you're doing some really odd things, or asking them to do some odd things, they wonder what on earth it's all about. Once I got comfortable with that, it was much better. **Sarah**

The GRBAS rating scale (Hirano, 1981) was also a very common assessment used. The scale is widely used in voice clinics around the UK to measure five aspects of voice quality: grade, roughness, breathiness, asthaenia and strain. The assessment allows clinicians to make a subjective judgement and award a rating for each aspect which can then be used to inform therapy and measure efficacy. In order to gain a comparable voice sample, most students asked their clients to read aloud a standard passage, most commonly the Rainbow Passage (Fairbanks, 1960). During the early stages of their placements, the students rated their client's voice using the GRBAS scale and compared their subjective judgements to those of their clinical educator's. As they gained experience of using this assessment, most of the students felt confident in making these judgements without the support of their CE. Some of the students also carried out rating scales and questionnaires to measure their client's levels of emotional stress. The results were then reviewed in the context of the case history and could be used to help explain to a client that high levels of stress could be causing or contributing to dysphonia.

Intervention

All five students gained experience of a range of direct and indirect intervention approaches and felt as though they gained a great deal of experience in terms of planning and carrying out therapy. Many commented that their clients did not know what to expect from a voice therapy session and that this was one of the major challenges of working with this client group.

> Most clients do think, "What on earth are you doing!"
> And I don't know what they expect when they come to

> a voice clinic…I don't think they know what to expect
> actually. I think they're really probably the client group
> that least knows why they're there or what can be done.
> They know their voice has changed, but that's about all
> their understanding is. **Sarah**

Several students found that, as students, there were some restrictions on the
range of direct therapy techniques that they were able to use because so many
require further postgraduate training. Nevertheless, the students generally
felt that their clinical skills developed during placement due to the highly
structured nature of the approaches they were using. Some were particularly
surprised at the fact they were using similar techniques to help people with
a wide range of diagnoses.

> I'd be getting bogged down in the details of the condition.
> But you could see clients with a variety of conditions
> and their end goal was still the same. To restore normal
> voice. **Sarah**

The students described a large number of techniques that they had used:
relaxation, breath support, humming, chewing (Froeschels, 1952), yawn–sigh
(Boone & McFarlane, 1993), deconstriction exercises and optimal pitch work
(Boone, 1983). Because of the range of unfamiliar techniques they were using,
the students spent lots of time reading up about the approaches in order to
increase their confidence and understanding.

> When you start asking them to chew, like chewing a big
> sticky toffee, you've got to be prepared, I think, so you feel
> expert enough, so you feel like you're not asking them to
> just do something stupid for the sake of it, and be prepared
> to explain, understand yourself and explain that to the
> client, in a way they can understand of course. I felt very
> uncomfortable at first but then I felt much more comfortable,
> because I'd done the reading. **Sarah**

Georgina and Rob both worked on desconstriction and relaxation exercises
with their clients who presented with psychogenic dysphonia. Intervention
techniques for psychogenic dysphonia vary upon the individual's needs and
therapist's skills. Although it can sometimes be resolved very quickly, in other
cases it can take an enormous amount of time and effort on the part of both the

therapist and the client (Baker, 1998) and encouraging clients to try particular techniques can be challenging.

> If they're not accepting that they have a psychological disorder they're not likely to embrace techniques such as relaxation. **Georgina**

Ann also experienced challenges in working with reluctant clients who felt self-conscious about carrying out some of the voice exercises. She helped her client to overcome these feelings by sharing her own stories to build rapport and help her client to relax. Feelings of embarrassment about performing the voice exercises were certainly not limited to the clients, though most students reported that these feelings reduced as they gained more experience of the techniques and began to feel more confident in their own abilities. Focusing on the client rather than themselves during these sessions was one of the most effective strategies.

> She [CE] was expecting me to join in straight away. It put the client at ease as well if we all did it. But I think it was on the second week only, I was sitting in her chair and I was kind of doing therapy with clients, which was great. I think ultimately when I look back, scary as that was at first, to be thrown in straight away, I think it was brilliant. There can be no substitute for just getting stuck in as soon as possible really, as scary as it is. And you'd like to put it off, but at the same time you know you should just throw yourself in. **Sarah**

Georgina worked closely with two clients, a singer and a male-to-female transsexual client, on obtaining optimal pitch using standard hierarchies of complexity (Boone, 1983). She found it especially difficult to provide accurate models for her clients and practised the techniques at home prior to her sessions to improve her own skills.

> I don't have a musical bone in my body and I suppose there's terminology associated with music such as pitch and range and things like that, but also there's the fact that I'm supposed to be modelling something to singers. I'm supposed to be doing a scale and I know that they're far better than me [even] with their voice disorder. So that's

> what I struggled with most, and I think it was overcoming
> that and just biting the bullet and thinking you've just got
> to do it. **Georgina**

The students all carried out some indirect intervention over the course of their placement, including voice rest, vocal hygiene and education. Indirect intervention is designed to address the psychosocial factors that can influence voice, such as occupation, social life, environmental factors and emotional status (Enderby et al., 2009a). A variety of techniques and strategies were employed to to address one or more of these areas depending on the circumstances of individual clients.

> It was getting them to think about how they could alleviate
> the areas of stress in their lives. Because you're kind of going,
> "Oh, this problem you're having in your life is causing you
> to have a problem somewhere else." It was difficult and that
> was where I was most heavily supported by my clinicians
> to try and do it in a gentle fashion. **Ann**

One of the most important clinical skills that the students developed was in helping their clients to understand how the voice works and the range of factors that can lead to dysphonia. Several students developed pictorial resources to aid their explanations and some used 3-dimensional models of the larynx to show their clients how the voice is produced. Nevertheless, this aspect of voice therapy proved to be one of the most difficult and also one of the most important factors in encouraging clients to carry out voice exercises at home.

> They sit at home thinking, "Why am I doing this again?"
> And it's easy for them to lose track of why they're doing it. I
> think with voice, it's much more difficult to understand that
> link than it is with recovering from a broken leg…we used
> to talk about how if you had a broken leg you wouldn't just
> run to start, you have to build up your exercise, build up
> your stamina, build up your muscles. And it's no different
> for your voice, you've got muscles in there that support your
> voice…and we need to work with all of that. You know, it's
> finding that way to explain. **Sarah**

Playing a role in their clients' recovery from dysphonia was one of the most rewarding aspects of these placements. The students felt that the degree of recovery was very heavily influenced in most cases by a client's attitude and their willingness to make lifestyle changes. One of the most important elements to the success of voice therapy was the level of motivation that clients had to practise techniques between sessions.

> People came back and said, "Actually, on the phone it was really great because my daughter could hear me." **Ann**

The improvement experienced by some clients was very rapid, something that pleased both the clients and the students, although on occasions such rapid recovery did make it difficult to plan sessions.

> Quite often you'd see someone one week and the next week they come back and say, "My voice is much better." **Rob**

In most instances, the fact that clients attended speech and language therapy meant they were motivated to follow the advice they were given. However, some of the students discovered that a small proportion of clients found it difficult to take specific advice on board, particularly if they felt that the recommended changes would have a detrimental impact on their daily lives. Rob worked with a sports coach who had suffered a vocal cord haemorrhage and was concerned about the impact of vocal rest on her ability to do her job effectively.

> The treatment for haemorrhage is complete voice rest, and she was like "I can't do it." I think that's the thing with a lot of voice things, you can [say], "This is the best thing to do, you can either do it and you get the best outcome, or you can not do it, and it's up to you." **Rob**

Summary

The students all felt that their clinical skills had developed significantly by the end of their placements and that their experience had helped them to develop a wide range of transferable skills. They felt particularly confident in terms of building rapport with clients, taking detailed case histories and working with people who may be emotionally vulnerable. Although voice is a particularly specialist area of speech and language therapy, the students felt as though they gained plenty of practical experience and were surprised about how much of their knowledge and skills they could transfer across client groups.

> I suppose I really liked the variety, I found the whole thing fascinating. So you had people who had diagnosed conditions or structural difficulties that caused the voice problem, but then you had the psychogenic element. **Sarah**

Top tips from students

- Be able to explain how a 'normal' voice works in a way that is accessible to clients.
- Be prepared for clients to ask lots of questions!
- Clients may be very emotional, especially some who have psychogenic dysphonia. Keep some tissues handy!
- Be thorough in your case history. Although clients may present with the same symptoms, the reasons may be very different from one another.
- Do some reading on the most common conditions before your placement starts. I found conditions such as reflux, psychogenic dysphonia and chronic obstructive pulmonary disease were very common.
- When you know which assessment or therapy you are going to do, practise at home! It's quite a fun thing. Who doesn't want to practise relaxation techniques!
- Think about which area each part of your case history form is gathering information about, e.g., functional, emotional, environmental.

Top tips from clinical educators

- Ensure that you have a basic understanding of how a normal voice works and understand the relationship between breathing and voicing.
- These patients can usually talk more than other client groups, so the ability to build rapport with a patient is fundamental...show that you are interested!
- Understand the effects of stress or emotional upset on the voice.
- Therapy plans are for your own confidence, but always be guided by the client.
- It is not possible to read up on everything about voice, but read in relation to the clients that you see so that your clinical experience will be meaningful.
- Don't be afraid to ask your CE lots of questions!

13 The future of clinical education

The preceding chapters have offered a unique insight into the real, lived experiences of clinical placements in speech and language therapy. Of course, these are the views of individual students and do not necessarily represent the experience of all students. Furthermore, not all types of placement have been covered in this book. As speech and language therapy services change, so too do the placements available to students. Keeping up with demand and offering students a wide range of experiences will continue to be a challenge that commissioners, universities and speech and language therapy services need to work together to address. It is hoped that this book provides potential and existing students with a greater understanding of the challenges and highlights of most placements they may encounter during their studies. In addition, the book provides an insight into the views and opinions of clinical educators from a wide range of specialist fields and may help students to gain a deeper understanding of what it expected of them whilst on placement.

This book delivers an honest account of the highs and the lows of being on placement. Almost every student was enthusiastic and inspired by their experiences, regardless of the client group they worked with and the type of placement they experienced. Having the opportunity to put their skills into practice and apply the knowledge that they had learned in the classroom was exciting and rewarding. Many of the students felt that long periods of studying between placements meant they sometimes lost sight of the profession they were working so hard to enter. Placements served as a reminder of the end goal: becoming a practising speech and language therapist.

From student to practising clinician

Becoming a newly-qualified speech and language therapist is an exciting yet daunting prospect. Although placements are often hard-work and stressful, students are well-supported by both academic staff and clinical supervisors. Their caseload is purposefully selected to be manageable yet stimulating. There is time to conduct detailed assessments, to write comprehensive session plans and to discuss clients often at great length. Even during their final placement, when most students have taken on a more autonomous role, they can turn to their clinical educator for support in making difficult decisions, safe in the knowledge that they will be guided and advised to work in the best interests of their client. At the end of each placement, students return to university to debrief and discuss their experiences with peers in a familiar environment.

Working as a newly-qualified therapist creates a whole host of new challenges in terms of time management, staff meetings and managing a caseload of clients, all in an unfamiliar environment with new colleagues. These are exciting times for new graduates, but the experience can be overwhelming at first. Most new graduates will spend the initial weeks of a new post at induction events, shadowing other therapists and meeting the team of professionals that they will be working alongside. There is also a formal support system in place in the UK to support new therapists during the early stages of their career. New graduates must register with the HCPC in order to practise as a speech and language therapist. Newly-qualified practitioners (NQPs) become supervised members of the RCSLT and must achieve the competencies outlined in the framework for NQPs before they are able to transfer to full membership of the RCSLT. Usually this process takes between 12 and 18 months and the SLT is expected to demonstrate competence in eight areas, including service improvement, personal and people development and communication.

Although not prescriptive, the RCSLT advises that a number of support systems are put in place to support and enhance development to enable autonomous practice. Weekly meetings with a line manager during the first three months are recommended, with monthly meetings for the remainder of the period as a NQP. Many new SLTs are also partnered with a mentor to support them with their everyday work. Research suggests that most NQPs receive some degree of support once in their first post (Brumfitt et al., 2005), though this varies in terms of whether this is achieved via formal meetings or more informal conversations about any arising issues. Once the competencies outlined in the NQP framework have been achieved, full autonomous membership of the RCSLT can be granted.

Many of the final year students in the present study were eager to secure their first post and felt ready to take this next step, whereas others remained anxious about whether they were sufficiently competent and lacked confidence in their abilities. These findings mirror previous research, which showed that 69% of NQPs felt confident about their skills upon graduation, but 31% still felt that they lacked self-confidence (Brumfitt et al., 2005). The same study also reported on the aspects of practice that came as a surprise to new graduates in their first post. Fifty-eight percent reported that organising their workload was the biggest shock, 39% were surprised by the number of clients on their caseload and 19% were shocked at the sense of responsibility that they felt once in post. Perhaps more encouragingly, the newly-qualified therapists felt that informal support from colleagues was invaluable and that their confidence in terms of working with clients gradually increased with time and experience (Brumfitt et al., 2005).

The future of clinical education

Clinical placements in speech and language therapy have remained relatively unchanged since the profession began. Most universities allocate one student to a practising speech and language therapist who will supervise the student's clinical practice on block (usually more than two days per week for a number of weeks) or weekly placements and provide guidance and support. In recent years, challenges to this traditional model have emerged and other options are being trialled and considered across the allied health professions at an international level. Changes to speech and language service structures, financial and staffing constraints and a general increase in the commissioned number of students have all contributed to a stretch in the allocation of suitable placements for students (Jones, Yeung, & Webb, 1998). Consequently, a range of alternative placement options is being considered to ease the pressure on both universities and service providers whilst maintaining high standards of supervision for students. A study of placement models used on speech pathology programmes in seven countries showed that a range of 'non-traditional' approaches such as interprofessional, specialist and project placements were being used in the UK, Australia and Canada (Sheepway, Lincoln, & Togher, 2011). Interprofessional placements are defined as students from different disciplines working and actively learning together, for instance, a speech pathology student working with a physiotherapy student on postural stability for swallowing. Project placements are used on some speech pathology courses in Australia, South Africa and the UK (Sheepway et al., 2011). They are a relatively new mode of clinical placement in speech and language therapy but have been used widely as a model of clinical education in occupational therapy (Prigg & Mackenzie, 2002). Students work on a project that has been set up for them by the speech and language therapy service they are placed with, for example trialling and evaluating a therapy approach or producing educational materials. Evaluation of project placements suggests that students develop professionals skills whilst the SLT department benefits from their input; however, students receive less supervision and, depending upon the project, may gain less experience of working with clients (Sheepway et al., 2011). Perhaps the most common non-traditional placements with the largest evidence-base are peer placements, where two or more students are allocated a single placement and clinical supervisor. Feedback from students on peer placements is often positive, with benefits including reduced stress, reassurance and learning from each other (Grundy, 2004). Certainly those students on peer placement interviewed for this book agreed that they gained a great deal from peer placements and felt that they benefitted enormously from the support and knowledge of their peer.

> I think we were just both quite excited to have a peer, because we both felt like at this stage, you don't know it all. She'd had a lot of adult experience in her previous placement, I'd had a lot of paediatric experience and so in that sense we complemented each other. We had some days together… one of them was head and neck cancer. Well, for me that was just really scary. I was really out of my comfort zone, but she was OK about it, and she was like, "Look, you're going to be all right on Tuesdays, I'm going to be all right on Fridays." We'd just support each other and it was fantastic, in fact we made friends…it's been great. I wouldn't say there was anything negative about it. A lot of the time we had to do peer feedback, so we had to watch each other doing sessions and give feedback to each other. You never wanted to say anything negative about each other. We always had to think of one thing that you'd do differently, and we both did that and we were both OK about it, because I just think you just wanted to take any feedback that you could and let it enhance the person that you are because you're never going to get everything right. And at the end of every week, she'd be like, "Has it been alright this week for you, is there anything that's upset you, have I annoyed you?" So we were both really reflective and very honest with each other. **Martina**

Emotional support was one of the greatest advantages highlighted by all the students on peer placements, irrespective of whether they knew their peer prior to the placement. One of the main concerns reported in the literature is that some students feel they may not receive sufficient individual attention from their clinical educator and that this may impact upon their final marks (Grundy, 2004). A small number of students in the present study touched upon these concerns, but felt that the advantages gained from peer placements vastly outweighed any downsides of their experience.

> It was very different to what I had done before. But actually having someone else there was really, really helpful. We could bounce ideas off each other, and if we were having a particularly hard day, you'd have someone who you [could talk to] and then just carry on with your day. We both had strengths in different areas as well, and I think that's a really good thing about peer placements because where my knowledge lacked hers excelled, and where mine excelled hers lacked. Sometimes feedback from my clinical educator could be a bit mixed because they were feeding back to two people who they amalgamated into one. So I might not have got as specific feedback as I would as an individual. **Ella**

The structure and form of clinical placements are gradually evolving in response to ongoing changes to healthcare provision, both at national and international levels. It is vital that students continue to receive excellent supervision and a wide range of experiences, but how these standards will continue to be met requires further research, specifically in the context of speech and language pathology.

Conclusion

This book provides a snapshot of how students feel and what they experience whilst on placement. The huge range of skills, knowledge and experiences recalled by the students goes some way towards illustrating the complexity and diversity of a career as a speech and language therapist. The results suggest that the stresses of clinical exams, the anxiety surrounding new experiences and the challenges of combining placement with endless academic work are all far outweighed by the rewards of working as part of a team that aims to improve another person's quality of life. Many of the students interviewed for this study commented on how much they enjoyed having the opportunity to reflect back on their placement in much more detail than they would do usually. Some found it cathartic, and others came to realise just how much they had learned through their experiences, good and bad. Perhaps all students should take a note of this and take a moment after each placement to reflect on all that they have learned and the progress that they are continually making. I have no doubt that the insight, knowledge and enthusiasm displayed by all of the students involved will lead them to long and rewarding careers as capable and confident speech and language therapists.

Acknowledgements

I would like to thank Hannah Johnston and Eve Lucas for their invaluable help and patience in transcribing the mountains of interview data. I am also very grateful to my colleagues at Manchester Metropolitan University for their encouragement and support. Thank you to my very dear proof reader, you know who you are. Finally, I would like to express my gratitude to Meaghan Reid, a former student at Manchester Metropolitan University. Talking to Meaghan about her fascinating experiences on placement sparked the initial idea for this book. She spoke with passion, insight and enormous sensitivity about her clients and I am sure she will go on to have the successful career that she deserves.

References

Adams, C., Cooke, R., Crutchley, A., Hesketh, A., & Reeves, D. (2001). *Assessment of Comprehension and Expression 6-11 (ACE)*. London: GL Assessment.

Adams, M. (1990). The demands and capacities model 1. *Journal of Fluency Disorders, 15*, 135–141.

Adamson, J., Beswick, A., & Ebrahim, S. (2004). Is stroke the most common cause of disability? *Journal of Stroke and Cerebrovascular Diseases, 12*, 171–177.

Armstrong, S. & Ainley, M. (2012). *South Tyneside Assessment of Phonology 2 (STAP)*. St Mabyn, UK: STASS Publications.

Attride-Stirling, J. (2001). Thematic networks: An analytic tool for qualitative research. *Qualitative Research, 1*, 385–405.

Baker, J. (1998). Psychogenic dysphonia: Peeling back the layers. *Journal of Voice, 12*(4), 527–535.

Bakheit, A.M., Shaw, S., Barrett, L., Wood, J., Carrington, S., Griffiths, S., et al. (2007). A prospective, randomised, parallel group controlled study of the effect of intensity of speech and language therapy on early recovery from post stroke aphasia. *Clinical Rehabilitation, 21*(10), 885–874.

Bishop, D. (2003). *Test for Reception of Grammar - 2*. Oxford: Pearson Assessment.

Bondy, A.S. & Frost, L.A. (1994). The Picture Exchange Communication System. *Focus on Autistic Behavior, 9*(3), 1–19.

Boone, D.R. (1983). *Voice and Voice Therapy* (Third edition ed.). London: Prentice-Hall.

Boone, D.R. & McFarlane, S.C. (1993). A critical view of the yawn–sigh as a voice therapy technique. *Journal of Voice, 7*(1), 75–80.

Botting, N., Crutchley, A., & Conti-Ramsden, G. (1998). Educational transitions of 7-year-old children with SLI in language units: A longitudinal study. *International Journal of Language & Communication Disorders, 33*(2), 177–219.

Bradshaw, J. (2007). Between you and me. In S. Carnaby (Ed.), *Learning Disability Today*. Brighton: Pavillion.

Broomfield, J. & Dodd, B. (2004). Children with speech and language disability: Caseload characteristics. *International Journal of Language & Communication Disorders, 39*, 1–22.

Brumfitt, S.M., Enderby, P., & Hoben, K. (2005). The tranistion to work of newly qualified speech and language therapists: Implications for the curriculum. *Learning in Health and Social Care, 4*(3), 142–155.

Bryan, A. (1997) Colourful semantics: Thematic role therapy. In S. Chiat, J. Law and

J. Marshall (Eds), *Language Disorders in Children and Adults: Psycholinguistic approaches to therapy*. London: Whurr.

Bryan, K. (2004). Prevalence of speech and language difficulties in young offenders. *International Journal of Language & Communication Disorders, 39*, 391–400.

Bryan, K., Freer, J., & Furlong, C. (2007). Language and communication difficulties in juvenile offenders. *International Journal of Language & Communication Disorders, 42*, 505–520.

Care Quality Commission. (2013). *Safeguarding Protocol.*

Carroll, K., Murad, S., Eliahoo, J., & Majeed, A. (2001). Stroke incidence and risk factors in a population-based prospective cohort study. *Health Statistics Quarterly, 12*(Winter).

Chamberlain, L., Chung, M.C., & Jenner, L. (1993). Preliminary findings on communication and challenging behaviour. *Learning Difficulty, 39*(2), 118–125.

Chan, J., Carter, S., & McAllister, L. (1994). Contributors to anxiety in clinical education in undergraduate speech-language pathology students. *Australian Journal of Human Communication Disorders, 22*(1), 57–73.

Chapman, K.L., Hardin-Jones, M.A., Schulte, J., & Halter, K.A. (2001). Vocal development of 9-month-old babies with cleft palate. *Journal of Speech, Language and Hearing Research, 44*, 1268–1283.

Chipchase, L.S., Buttrum, P.J., Dunwoodie, R., Hill, A.E., Mandrusiak, A., & Moran, M. (2012). Characteristics of student preparedness for clinical learning: Clinical educator perspectives using the Delphi approach. *BMC Medical Education, 12*, 112.

Christie, J., Clark, W., & Mortenson, L. (1986). *Mount Wilga High Level Language Test.* Sydney: Mount Wilga Rehabilitation Centre.

Clegg, J., Hollis, C., & Rutter, M. (1999). Life sentence. *RCSLT Bulletin, 571*, 16–18.

Constantinidou, G., Wertheimer, J.C., Tsandis, J., Evan, C., & Paul, D.R. (2012). Assessment of executive functioning in brain injury: Collaboration between speech-language pathology and neuropsychology for an integrative neuropsychological perspective. *Brain Injury, 26*(13–14), 1549–1563.

Crawford, E. & Bull, R. (2006). Teenagers' difficulties with keywords regarding the criminal court process. *Psychology, Crime and Law, 12*(6), 654–667.

Crew, M. & Ellis, N. (2008). *Speech and language therapy within Bradford Youth Offending Team: Report outlining the findings of a six-month pilot project examining the speech and language needs of the clients within Bradford Youth Offending Team.* Bradford: Bradford Youth Offending Team.

Crichton-Smith, I. (2002). Communicating in the real world: Accounts from people who stammer. *Journal of Fluency Disorders, 27*, 333–352.

Csefalvay, Z., Hansson, K., Wigforss, E., Patterson, A., Peleman, M., Stansfield, J., et al.

(2013). *NetQues Project Report. Speech and Language Therapy Education in Europe. United in Diversity.*

Cummins, J. (2000). *Language, Power and Pedagogy; Bilingual children in the crossfire.* Clevedon: Mutlilingual Matters Ltd.

Dabul, B. (2000). *Apraxia Battery for Adults (ABA-2)* (Second edition ed.). Austin, Tx.: PRO-ED, Inc.

Deary, I.J., Wilson, J.A., Carding, P.N., & Mackenzie, K. (2003). The dysphonic voice heard by me, you and it: Differential associations with personality and psychological distress. *Clinical Otolaryngology, 28*, 374–378.

Demmink-Geertman, L. & Dejonckere, P.H. (2002). Nonorganic habitual dysphonia and autonomic dysfunction. *Journal of Voice, 16*, 549–559.

Department for Education and Skills. (2001). *Special Educational Needs Code of Practice.* London.

Department of Health. (1998). *Signposts for Success in Commissioning and Providing Health Services for People with Learning Disabilities.* London.

Department of Health. (2004). *Better Health in Old Age.* London.

Department of Health. (2009). *Valuing People Now, Summary Report.* London.

Dilbert, C. & Goldenberg, D. (1995). Preceptors' perceptions of benefits, rewards, supports and commitment to preceptor role. *Journal of Advanced Nursing, 21*, 1144–1151.

Dodd, B., Hua, Z., Crosbie, S., Holm, A., & Ozanne, A. (2006). *Diagnostic Evaluation of Articulation and Phonology (DEAP).* London, UK: Pearson Assessment.

Dunn, L.M., Dunn, D.M., Sewell, J., Styles, B., Bryzyska, B., Shamson, Y., et al. (2009). *British Picture Vocabulary Scales-3 (BPVS-3).* London: GL Assessment Limited.

Elks, L. & McLachlan, H. (2007). *Test of Abstract Language Comprehension (TALC).* St Mabyn, Cornwall.

Enderby, P. (1996). *Stammering: What research is telling us.* British Stammering Association.

Enderby, P. & Emerson, J. (1995). *Does Speech and Language Therapy Work?* London: Whurr.

Enderby, P. & Palmer, R. (2008). *Frenchay Dysarthria Assessment (FDA-2)* (Second edition ed.). Austin, Tx.: PRO-ED, Inc.

Enderby, P., Pickstone, C., John, A., Fryer, K., Cantrell, A., & Papaioannou, D. (2009a). *RCSLT Resource Manual for Commissioning and Planning Services for SCLN: Voice.* London: RCSLT.

Enderby, P., Pickstone, C., John, A., Fryer, K., Cantrell, A., & Papaioannou, D. (2009b). *RCSLT Resource Manual for Commissioning and Planning Services for SLCN: Autistic Spectrum Disorders.* London: RCSLT.

Enderby, P., Pickstone, C., John, A., Fryer, K., Cantrell, A., & Papaioannou, D. (2009c). *RCSLT Resource Manual for Commissioning and Planning Services for SLCN: Cleft Lip/Palate and Velopharyngeal Impairment.* London: RSCLT.

Enderby, P., Pickstone, C., John, A., Fryer, K., Cantrell, A., & Papaioannou, D. (2009d). *RCSLT Resource Manual for Commissioning and Planning Services for SLCN: Fluency.* London: RCSLT.

Enderby, P., Pickstone, C., John, A., Fryer, K., Cantrell, A., & Papaioannou, D. (2009e). *RSCLT Resource Manual for Commissioning and Planning Services for SLCN: Learning Disability.* London: RCSLT.

Enderby, P., Wood, V., & Wade, D. (2006). *Frenchay Aphasia Screening Test (FAST)* (Second ed.). New Jersey, US: Wiley-Blackwell.

Fairbanks, G. (1960). *Voice and Articulation Drillbook* (Second ed.). New York: Harper & Row.

Fergusson, D.M., Horwood, J., & Ridder, E. (2005). Show me the child at seven: The consequences of conduct problems in childhood for psychosocial functioning in adulthood. *Journal of Child Psychology and Psychiatry, 46*, 837–849.

Finch, E., Fleming, J., Brown, K., Lethlean, J., Cameron, A., & McPhail, S. (2013). The confidence of speech-language pathology students regarding communicating with people with aphasia. *BMC Medical Education, 13*(92).

Froeschels, E. (1952). Chewing method as therapy. *Archives of Otolaryngology, 56*, 427–434.

Frost, L.A. & Bondy, A.S. (1994). *The Picture Exchange Communication System Training Manual.* Cherry Hill, NJ: Pyramid Educational Consultants.

Gallagher, E.R. & Berg, J. (2012). Clinical correlate: Cleft lip and palate. In L.K. McCauley & M.J. Somerman (Eds), *Mineralized Tissues in Oral and Craniofacial Science: Biological principles and clinical correlates.* Ames, Iowa: John Wiley & Sons Inc.

Garrard, P., Bradshaw, D., Jager, H.R., Thompson, A.J., Losseff, N., & Playford, D. (2002). Cognitive dysfunction after isolated brain stem insult. An underdiagnosed cause of long term morbidity. *Journal of Neurology, Neurosurgery and Psychiatry, 73*, 191–194.

Garrett, M.F. (1988). Processes in language production. In F.I. Newmeyer (Ed.), *Linguistics: The Cambridge Survey: Ill. Language: Psychological and biological aspects.* Cambridge: Cambridge University Press.

Goldbart, J. & Caton, S. (2010). *Communication and People with the Most Complex Needs: What works and why is this essential.* London: Mencap.

Grundy, K. (2004). Peer placements. In S.M. Brumfitt (Ed.), *Innovations in Professional Education for Speech and Language Therapy.* London: Whurr Publishers Ltd.

Hamilton, J. (1999). *Speech, Language and Communication Therapy: A perspective from HMYOI Polmont. Internal Report.* Forth Valley Primary Care NHS Trust.

Health Protection Agency. (2009). *Clostridium difficile factsheet*. London: Health Protection Agency.

Heritage, M., Virag, G., & McCuaig, L. (2011). *Better Outcomes for Young Offenders. Exploring the impact of speech and language therapy in Youth Offending Teams in Derbyshire*.

Hirano, M. (1981). Psycho-acoustic evaluation of voice: GRBAS Scale for evaluating the hoarse voice. *Clinical Examination of Voice*. London: Springer.

HM Government. (2002). *Education Act*. London: HMSO.

HM Government. (2008). *Youth Crime Action Plan*. London: HMSO.

HM Government. (1998). *Crime and Disorder Act (c.37)*. London: HMSO.

Howard, S. & Lohmander, A. (Eds). (2011). *Cleft Palate Speech: Assessment and intervention*. Chichester: Wiley-Blackwell.

Humber, E. & Snow, P. C. (2001). The oral language skills of juvenile offenders: A pilot investigation. *Psychiatry, Psychology and Law, 8*, 1–11.

Joint Accreditation Committee of the Health Professions Council and Royal College of Speech and Language Therapists. (2002). *Guidelines on the Accreditation of Courses Leading to a Qualification in Speech and Language Therapy*. London.

Jones, A., Yeung, E., & Webb, C. (1998). Tripartite involvement in healthcare clinical education. *Journal of Allied Health, 27*, 97–102.

Jones, M., Onslow, M., Packman, A., Williams, S., Ormond, T., Schwartz, I., et al. (2005). Randomised control trial of the Limcombe programme of early stuttering intervention. *British Medical Journal (Clinical Research Edition), 331*.

Kaplan, E., Goodglass, H., & Weintraub, S. (1983). *Boston Naming Test (BNT)*. Philadelphia: Lea & Febiger.

Kay, J., Coltheart, M., & Lesser, R. (1992). *Psycholinguistic Assessments of Language Processing in Aphasia (PALPA)*. Hove, East Sussex: Psychology Press.

Keeling, M. & Keeling, K. (2006). *CLEAR: Phonology screening assessment*. Splisby: CLEAR Resources.

Kertesz, A. & McCabe, P. (1977). Recovery patterns and prognosis in aphasia. *Brain, 100*, 1–18.

Klein, J.F. & Hood, S.B. (2004). The impact of stuttering on employment opportunities and job performance. *Journal of Fluency Disorders, 29*, 255–273.

Kummer, A.W. (2008). *Cleft Palate and Craniofacial Anomalies: Effects on speech and resonance*. New York: Delmar Cengage Learning.

Laska, A.C., Hellblom, A., Murray, V., Kahan, T., & Von Arbin, M. (2001). Aphasia in acute stroke and relation to outcome. *Journal of Internal Medicine, 249*(5), 413–422.

Leow, A.M. & Lo, L.J. (2008). Palatoplasty: Evolution and controversies. *Chang Gung Medical Journal, 31*, 335–344.

Linares-Omara, N. (2005). Language-learning disorders and youth incarceration. *Journal of Communication Disorders, 38,* 311–319.

London Dysmorphology Database. from http://lmdatabases.com/about_lmd.html

Lord, C., Rutter, M., DiLavore, P.C., Risi, S., Gotham, K., & Bishop, S.L. (2012). *Autism Diagnostic Observation Schedule-2 (ADOS-2).* Torrance, CA.: Western Psychological Services.

Lowe, M. & Costello, A.J. (1988). *The Symbolic Play Test* (Second ed.). London, UK: GL Assessment Ltd.

Maguire, G., Riley, G., Wu, J., Franklin, D., & Potkin, S. (1997). PET scan evidence of parallel cerebral systems related to treatment effects: Effects of risperidone in the treatment of stuttering. In W. Hulstijn, H.F.M. Peters & P. H.H.M. van Lieshout (Eds), *International Congress Series 1146* (pp. 379–382). Amsterdam: Excerpta Medical.

Mann, G., Hankey, G., & Cameron, D. (1999). Swallowing function after stroke: Prognosis and prognostic factors at 6 months. *Stroke, 30,* 744–748.

Martino, R., Foley, N., Bhogal, S., Diamant, N., Speechley, M., & Teasell, R. (2005). Dysphagia after stroke: Incidence, diagnosis and pulmonary complications. *Stroke, 36*(12), 2756–2763.

Mathieson, L. (2001). *The Voice and its Disorders.* London: Whurr.

McAllister, L. & Lincoln, M. (2004). *Clinical Education in Speech-Language Pathology.* London: Whurr.

McAllister, L., Lincoln, M., McLeod, S., & Maloney, D. (1997). *Facilitating Learning in Clinical Settings.* Cheltenham: Stanley Thomas.

Menon, D.K., Schwab, K., Wright, D.W., & Maas, A.I. (2010). Position statement: Definition of traumatic brain injury. *Archives of Physical Medicine and Rehabilitation, 91*(11), 1637–1640.

Money, D. (2002). *Speech and Language Therapy Management Models in Management of Communication Needs in People with Learning Disabilities.* London: Whurr.

Morris, S.E. & Klein, M.D. (2000). *Pre-Feeding Skills: A comprehensive resource for mealtime development* (Second ed.). USA: Psychological Corporation.

Mossey, P. & Castillia, E. (2003). *Global Registry and Database on Craniofacial Anomalies.* Geneva: World Health Organisation Human Genetics Programme.

Mossey, P., Little, J., Munger, R.G., Dixon, M.J., & Shaw, W.C. (2009). Cleft lip and palate. *The Lancet, 374,* 1773–1785.

Nacro. (2011). *Speech, Language and Ccommunication Difficulties: Young people in trouble with the law.* London: Nacro.

National Institute for Health and Care Excellence. (2008). *NICE Clinical Guideline 68: Stroke: Diagnosis and initial management of acute stroke and transient ischaemic attack.* London: National Institute for Health and Clinical Excellence.

National Patient Safety Agency. (2004). *Understanding the patient safety issues for people with learning disabilities*. London.

Nind, M. & Hewett, D. (1988). Interaction as curriculum: A process method in a school for pupils with severe learning difficulties. *British Journal of Special Education, 15*, 55–57.

Nind, M. & Hewett, D. (1994). *Access to Communication: Developing the basics of communication with people with severe learning difficulties through Intensive Interaction.* London: David Fulton.

Onslow, M., Packman, A., & Harrison, E. (2003). *The Lidcombe Program of Early Stuttering Intervention: A clinician's guide*. Austin, TX: Pro-Ed.

Patterson, K. & Shewell, C. (1987). Speak and spell: Dissociations and word-class effects. In M. Coltheart, R. Job & G. Sartori (Eds), *The Cognitive Neuropsychology of Language*. Hillsdale, NJ: Lawrence Erlbaum.

Peterson-Falzone, S.J., Hardin-Jones, M.A., & Karnell, M.P. (2010). *Cleft Palate Speech* (4th edition). Philadelphia: Mosby.

Petheram, B. & Enderby, P. (2001). Demographic and epidemiological analysis of patients referred to speech and language therapy at eleven centres 1987–95. *International Journal of Language & Communication Disorders, 36*(4), 515–525.

Powell, T. (2004). *Head Injury: A practical guide*. Oxford: Headway and Winslow Press.

Prigg, A. & Mackenzie, L. (2002). Project placements for undergraduate occupational therapy students: Design, implementation and evaluation. *Occupational Therapy International, 9*, 210–236.

Qualifications and Curriculum Authority. (2009). *The P Scales*.

Renfrew, C. (2003). *The Renfrew Action Picture Test*. Oxford: Speechmark Publishing.

Rimmel, R.W., Jane, J.A., & Bond, M.R. (1990). Characteristics of the head injured patient. In M. Rosenthal, E.R. Griffith, M.R. Bond & J.D. Miller (Eds), *Cognitive Rehabilitation for Persons with Traumatic Brain Injury: A functional approach*. Baltimore, MD: Paul. H. Brookes.

Robertson, S.J. (1982). *Robertson Dysarthria Profile*. London: Robertson.

Roy, N., Stemple, J., Merrill, R., & Thomas, L. (2005). Voice disorders in the general population: Prevalence, risk factors and occupational impact. *The Laryngoscope, 115*(11), 1988–1995.

Royal College of Speech and Language Therapists. (1999). *Dysphagia Working Group: Recommendations for pre- and post-registration education and training*. London: RCSLT.

Royal College of Speech and Language Therapists. (2006). *Communicating Quality 3*. London: RCSLT.

Royal College of Speech and Language Therapists. (2007). *Good Practice for Speech and Language Therapists Working with Clients from Linguistic Minority Communities*. London: RCSLT.

Royal College of Speech and Language Therapists. (2009). *Locked Up and Locked Out: Communication is the key*. London: RSCLT.

Royal College of Speech and Language Therapists. (2010). *Position Paper: Adults with learning disabilities*. London.

Royal College of Speech and Language Therapists. (2012). *Speech, Language and Communication Needs in the Criminal Justice System and Best Practice Responses to These*. London: RCSLT.

Royal Hospital of Neurodisability. (2001). *Submission to Health Select Committee Inquiry into Head Injury: Rehabilitation*. Unpublished manuscript.

Rustin, L. (1987). *Assessment and Therapy Programme for Dysfluent Children*. Windsor: NFRE-Nelson.

Rustin, L., Botterill, W., & Kelman, E. (1996). *Assessment and Therapy for Young Dysfluent Children: Family interaction*. London: Whurr.

Schopler, E. & Reichler, R. (1964). *Treatment and Education of Autistic and Related Communication Handicapped Children*. Chapel Hill, NC: University of North Carolina.

Sell, D., Harding, A., & Grunwell, P. (1994). A screening assessment of cleft palate speech (Great Ormond Street Speech Assessment). *European Journal of Disorders of Communication, 29*, 1–15.

Semmel, E., Wiig, E.H., & Secord, W. (2006a). *Clinical Evaluation of Language Fundamentals Pre-school 2 UK (CELF2)*. London, UK: Pearson Assessment.

Semmel, E., Wiig, E.H., & Secord, W. (2006b). *Clinical Evaluation of Language Fundamentals-4 (CELF4)*. London: Pearson Assessment.

Sheepway, L., Lincoln, M., & Togher, L. (2011). An international study of clinical education practices in speech-language pathology. *International Journal of Speech-Language Pathology, 13*(2), 174–185.

Shiel, A., Wilson, B.A., McLellan, L., Watson, M., & Horn, S. (2000). *Wessex Head Injury Matrix*. London: Pearson.

Smith, E., Lemke, J., Taylor, M., Kirchner, L., & Hoffman, H. (1998). Frequency of voice problems among teachers and other occupations. *Journal of Voice, 12*, 480–488.

Snow, P.C., & Powell, M.B. (2005). What's the story? An exploration of narrative language abilities in male juvenile offenders. *Psychology, Crime and Law, 11*(3), 239–253.

Speech Pathology Australia. (2011). *Competency-based Occupational Standards for Speech Pathology Entry Level-Revised*.

Stackhouse, J. & Wells, B. (1997). *Children's Speech and Literacy Difficulties: A psycholinguistic framework*. London: Whurr.

Stansfield, J. (2004). Education for competent clinical practice. In S.M. Brumfitt (Ed.), *Innovations for Professional Education for Speech and Language Therapy*. London: Whurr.

Starkweather, C.W. (1987). *Fluency and Stuttering*. Englewood Cliffs, NJ: Prentice-Hall.

Swinburn, K., Porter, G., & Howard, D. (2004). *Comprehensive Aphasia Test (CAT)*. Hove, UK: Psychology Press.

Talbot, J. (2010). *Seen and Heard: Supporting vulnerable children in the youth justice system*. London: Prison Reform Trust.

Talbot, J. & Jacobsen, J. (2009). *Vulnerable Defendants in Criminal Court*. London: Prison Reform Trust.

Tate, R.L., Pfaff, A., Baguley, I.J., Marosszeky, J.E., Gurka, J.A., Hodgkinson, A.E., et al. (2006). A multicentre, randomised trial examining the effect of test procedures measuring emergence from post-traumatic amnesia. *Journal of Neurology, Neurosurgery and Psychiatry*, 77, 841–849.

The Foundation for People with Learning Disabilities. (2000). *Learning Disabilities: The fundamental facts*. London: The Foundation for People with Learning Disabilities.

The Hanen Centre. www.hanen.org.

Toppelberg, C.O., Tabors, P., Coggins, A., Lum, K., & Burger, C. (2005). Differential diagnosis of selective mutism in bilingual children. *Journal of the American Academy of Child and Adolescent Psychiatry*, 44(6), 592–595.

Trost-Cardamone, J.E. (1990). The development of speech: Assessing cleft palate misarticulations. In D.E. Kernahan & S.W. Rosenstein (Eds), *Cleft Lip and Palate: A system of management*. Baltimore: Williams & Wilkins.

van der Gaag, A., Smith, L., Davis, S., Moss, B., Cornelius, V., Laing, S., et al. (2005). Therapy and support services for people with long term stroke and aphasia and their relatives: A six month follow-up study. *Clinical Rehabilitation*, 19, 372.

Walker, M. (1978). The Makaton Vocabulary. In T. Tebbs (Ed.), *Ways and Means*. Basingstoke, UK: Globe.

Watkins, K., Smith, S., Davis, S., & Howell, P. (2005). Structural and functional abnormalities of the motor system in developmental stuttering. *Brain*, 131(1), 50–59.

Winter, K. (1999). Speech and language therapy provision for bilingual children: Aspects of the current service. *International Journal of Language & Communication Disorders*, 34(1), 85–98.

World Health Organisation. (1994). *International Classification of Diseases Tenth Edition (ICD-10) Mental and Behavioural Disorders*. Geneva: World Health Organisation.

World Health Organisation Human Genetics Programme. (2002). Global strategies to reduce the health-care burden of craniofacial anomalies: Report of WHO meetings on international collaborative research on craniofacial abnormalities. Geneva: World Health Organisation.

Wright, L. & Ayre, A. (2000). *Wright and Ayre Stuttering Self-Rating Profile*. Bicester: Winslow Press.

www.autism.org.uk/earlybird.

Index